THE LOVE OF A FATHER, A MOTHER AND A SON

BY

R GEORGE RIGGON

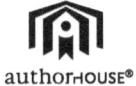

authorHOUSE®

AuthorHouse™ UK Ltd.
500 Avebury Boulevard
Central Milton Keynes, MK9 2BE
www.authorhouse.co.uk
Phone: 08001974150

First published by AuthorHouse 9/8/2007

ISBN: 978-1-4343-2171-8 (sc)

Printed in the United States of America
Bloomington, Indiana

This book is printed on acid-free paper.

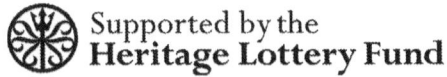

Supported by the
Heritage Lottery Fund

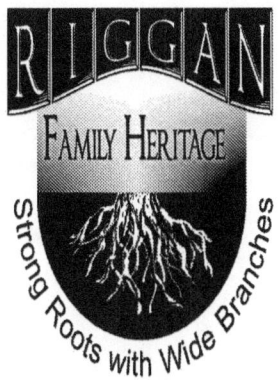

2007ricky@riggon01.wanadoo.co.uk

www.r-georgeriggon.com

Contents

Acknowledgement and Dedication

This book is dedicated to the memory of Sybil Eliza, Vandley Mark and Roland Riggan. During the respective but too short a time with us they had each made positive lasting contributions to the lives of many who are still alive today and are able to read this book. The precious memories they left behind are more than enough to sustain our love and unity as a family. May God continue to guide and protect all of our family in Africa, Jamaica, Britain, America, Canada and elsewhere that we have gone to work and live.

"In this day and age, families such as the Riggan's are very rare. Reading through this manuscript underscores my long held belief of their strength, integrity and closeness. They are a warm family, and I have felt accepted and loved from the beginning of our contact. Angie and I are, and will always be, proud to be part of the Riggan family. They are part of Vandley, whom we all loved and missed. Angie has a right to feel proud of her heritage from two different races and cultures, the Riggan and Eubanks families, yet bound in love and respect. My deepest thanks to Ricky for his time and hard work in putting together this rich and enlightening book."

(Susan Riggan, Charlotte, North Carolina, USA).

There is no greater love than the love you receive from God and that which you give to your family.

Family Love.
R. George Riggon
August 2007

Chapter One

The Matriarch

Younger children followed the lead of older sisters and brothers in referring to their parents as 'Aunt Lize' and 'Ron'. They were both born and raised in neighbouring rural districts in the western parish of Hanover in Jamaica. Their early childhood in the mid to late 1920s left them exposed to material hardship on the island during the height of British colonial rule in much of the Caribbean. Ron's father, Samuel Riggan had married his mother Margaret 'Argag' Moodie around the beginning of the 1900s. They amassed a total of sixteen children together while Samuel added at least one other child to his personal tally. The life they lead was very much in keeping with that past era when freedom from slavery was quickly replaced by the control of European nations. Working to survive from day to day was the highest priority for the families of ex-slaves on the island.

The ability to read and write was the preserve of the white settlers who ruled the island and took control over all its natural assets. A small window of an opportunity to gain the basics of literacy and numeracy was left open for a trickle of black people to work at the bottom of the chain as Christian missionaries, nurses, policing and plantation workers.

Lize took better advantage of the very limited opportunity for reading and writing that was available to black people on the island under the rule of Britain. The provision of basic education was organised through church missions such as those established by Anglicans, Roman Catholic, Methodist, Quaker, Baptist and Presbyterian. Attendance at school was not compulsory and would end by the age of twelve. Lize started her basic schooling at around seven years old. She was a very keen student who developed the ability to read and write very well from an early age. Her father provided her with the slates and chalk used to practice writing. The school uniform was a prized possession to be cared for and kept intact for the 'hand me down' to the next sibling in the family. The children listened to teachers reading books about England and about the glorious history of conquests by its great kings and queens.

The contrast in elementary schooling experience between the girl Lize and the boy Ron could not be further apart. Ron never learned to read or write and allayed the blame to this on his early responsibility to contribute to the upkeep of the family from an early age. Ron did not foresee a future requirement for reading and writing. Within families of ten and more children the experience of colonial education was very similar. Without the focus on a future that required reading and writing skills, the young Ron and his peers conceived of themselves only as inheriting the past of their own parents. A working life would be spread between the paid seasonal labour on agricultural farms and commercial plantations, and in providing unskilled manual labour to the emerging industries of building, lumber, stone and roadwork. Only a small minority of black children would fulfil ambitions to receive training for positions in service to white colonial settlers and Asian administrators. Migrant Arab and Jewish communities were also higher placed in the hierarchy of colour and wealth.

When Lize came to the end of her time at Brownsville Elementary School in Cascade, she had reached the age of twelve. The first ambition she expressed about future work was familiar enough. She had always been numerate and highly literate with early signs of a willingness to assist others within her family. The task of reading letters received by her father fell to her from an early age. Samuel Patterson would say the words to his letters of reply while Lize translate them into written English. The white head teacher had seen the potential in young Lize during her five years at Brownsville elementary school in Cascade. He was aware that the black subjects of the British colony were restricted to work in menial and unskilled work. The racial hierarchy of the island would eventually encouraged a small number of 'brown coloured' black people into some areas of public service as the population continued to increase and expand across the island. Lize recognised the futility of holding any lofty ambition and on the advice of her father, she settled for something that was more in line with the realistic expectation for a young black woman on the island prior to the 1960s.

Lize started a period of apprenticeship with a well-known dressmaker in the parish capital of Lucea. Mrs Conner was the second or third generation of seamstress in her family. The family were brown skinned and they owned local clothes stores, land, and the building hosting the post office in the district. They were rich people by the standard of the time.

"You can read and write?" Mrs Conner enquired from the tall brown skinned girl.

"Yes ma'am", was the reply from Lize, as she maintained a look of self-confidence. The manner of her speech and tone was mature. Mrs Conner could see that the young woman was from a family background that was similar to her own, at least in terms of the tone of the skin. She observed the well-kept sheen

3

in the plaited black hair. The straight nose gave the long angular face a touch of attractiveness. The well-ironed light coloured blouse was tucked neatly into dark skirts that fell below the roll of the knees. The shiny opened-toed shoes were purchased only recently to replace the pair made rugged and scuffed by Sunday school.

"You ever used a sewing machine before?". Mrs Conner continued without waiting for the words that she was certain to follow the firm instant nod of the young woman's head. She would have noted the impatience in the light brown eyes of the young Lize Patterson.

"If you break any of the machines I will have to take back the money out of the three shillings a week what I pay you. You understand?"

"I understand, ma'am, and I will be very careful with your machine". Lize followed the heavy seamstress to the vacant seat at a biscuit coloured Singer sewing machine positioned to the left of two other machines. Another young woman who was unknown to Lize was paying studious attention to the garment under the machine in front of her. She did not look up as Mrs Conner walked by while giving Lize her instructions about the time of work and level of effort expected.

In this environment the only authority was Mrs Conner. She determined the terms of work and every young woman who came to train under her was left with no doubt about the matter. It was her who had the power to give these unskilled and as yet untrained black girls the opportunity to make something of their lives and in her eyes, they should be grateful. Each young woman soon became aware that in order to please Mrs Conner they would be required to demonstrate good discipline of hard work and ambition. For some of them there would then be the hope of a permanent job and the prospect to earn and save some money before a husband came along. A husband from a good family could be a decisive step to a prosperous life like that of Mrs Conner's.

The period of an informal apprenticeship for a seamstress could last up to two or three years. Much would depend on the speed at which a young woman was able to learn the craft of her trade. It could also depend on the personal favour of the proprietor to the trainees. If an offer of a job came along in the meantime or, if for any other reason the trainee moved away from the local area, the period of tenure would be ended. By the end of her time with Mrs Conner, Lize had learned the craft of an apprentice seamstress. She had lived with her father and stepmother and older sisters, Olive and Dorcas from the age of two. Her mother Estry had another family with her own husband and was also living in the district of Cascade. A badly damaged foot sustained while labouring on a plantation had left her father disabled. The damage was severe and the affected leg was eventually amputated. For the entirety of her young life, Lize cared for her father without complaint or murmur.

As part of the contribution she made to the household, Lize was already well practised in hand sewing with needles and thread. In time she would supplement the income of her own young family by taking on jobs of sewing and dressmaking through contacts of family and friends. The end of the apprenticeship under Mrs Connor was hastened to an end following an incident that had occurred with the husband of the seamstress. He had developed quite a fancy for a number of the young women in training. He would make promises of permanent work to the young apprentices. When he turned his attention to the attractive young Lize, she let the man of more than three times her age know in no uncertain terms that she was not interested in his favours.

"Mr Connor, you a big man fe me and me naa look fe nobody. So a beg you to leave me alone, sir."

When he persisted, she was very direct with her threat to bring the matter to the attention of Mrs Connor. Since his respectability-conscious wife would not be inclined to uphold the complaint of her young apprentice Lize felt that her only viable option was to leave voluntarily.

It was through her older sister Dorcas that Lize met Ron around the time of 1940. He lived in the neighbouring district of Montpelier. The former sugarcane and banana plantations worked by slaves on the estates of Tryall and Maggotty were near to the district of Cascade, and these provided the only real opportunity for young men to find manual farm labour. Their relationship developed over the following months and when they agreed to set-up a home together, it was Ron who opted to migrate from Montpelier to the district of Cascade. But before making the move Ron had to ponder whether he should really leave the nest of his own family. He knew that Lize was very close to her father and would not think of deserting him. She told him of her relationship with Ron and of his intention that they should live together. Samuel was not sure.

"But a who is this boy who want to come ya and tek 'way me daughter?" He didn't pause for the reply.

The old man continued, "Me want to know a who him, and see if is good somebody."

Lize attempted to provide him with her own reassurance, "Me father, them name Riggan and them come from over Mompelier."

"Mom-pelier? The old man's accent echoed to the mispronounced name of the district.

"But me think me know the fam-bly? A who a fe him father?"

"Him father name Mass Sammy Riggan. You and them used to work a Moggotty", replied Lize.

Samuel interrupted.

"Out a Maggotty Bush?"

"Yes, me father."

"Well me think me know them. The Riggan breed them a no bad people. But a nuff brothers a them."

He was nearly content on the matter, "But carry him come, make a get fe talk to him and find out him intention fe you."

Samuel Patterson was advanced in years and had become hard of hearing. He had established the young man's family and that was very important to him. He had now signalled his intention to fulfil a final duty on behalf of his highly favoured daughter. He had reared her from a young age and he wanted to be assured that she was going into a good family. He had his own land and he walked slowly from the house to show a spot to his daughter.

"Me tell them say when you ready, you can build one house right there so."

He gestured with a finger to the exact area of land.

"A fe you spot that. Me give it to you."

Lize surveyed the small area and she could already imagine the shape and size of her first house together with her future husband and family.

The house they built was made out of thatched material stripped from trees and plotted with pieces of wood to the sides. The roof was covered with zinc and straw. There was no building blocks or bricks or mortar. Only great estate buildings could afford those materials. The black poor on the island would be quite satisfied to erect a home of sticks and straw. When the roof and sides were covered and secured they would maintain a dry earth base by digging deep trenches around the perimeter of the house as a means by which to control the flow and draining of rainwater. The protective material overhanging the roof extended sufficiently to nullify the penetration of water falling too close to the base or immediate surrounds of the small house. Their four oldest children Bibs, Ken, Earva and brother

Vandley were born in Cascade at intervals of roughly two years apart from 1943 to 1950.

Those years were hard times for Lize and Ron but they made a success of their early life together. They were both determined to provide their young family with security and so they utilised the small plot of land to grow their our own food. They cultivated corn, peas, yam, banana and sorrel. There were also breadfruit and mango. Lize was especially pleased that Ron's parents, Samuel and Argag, also offered their full blessing and approval to the future bride of their fifth son.

Lize and Ron relocated from Cascade to live near the nest of the Riggan family in Montpelier district after getting married in August 1950. That was a year after the death of her father and marked the beginning of an irrevocable dispute with her father's remaining children and widow over entitlement and ownership of the land he had left behind. The episode stirred deep emotions of anger and resentment in Lize. But rather than engage in daily quarrels with her siblings, she would leave her inheritance behind. That spirit of determination and independence drove her life choices and decisions in future years. The move to Montpelier led to the ambition to purchase their own land and secure a future for their young family. After the next three children arrived in Montpelier in the years between 1951 and 1956 a new era for the island was set in motion.

Following the years of war between the main British and European powers, and including the later participation of America and Japan, the rate of popular unemployment soared. As an outlet, many youth on the island took up the opportunity to sell their labour overseas through seasonal manual work on American sugar cane, apples, orange and cotton plantations. The labour shortage that occurred in Britain, Europe and North

America after the Second World War effectively created the conditions for labour migration between the island and British and North American industrialising cities. Ron was reluctant to consider any such venture into unknown foreign territories. He had learned on the island about the hostile treatment of black people in the deep south of America. He had heard by hear say about the harsh treatment of foreign workers on American farms and plantations.

Domestic and overseas employment opportunity on the island had fallen away with the reduction in the agricultural export markets in Western Europe and North America. Experience of life on the island in the years following the war years was quite harsh for the growing black population in the rural agricultural parishes of Hanover, Westmoreland, Trelawny, St Anns and elsewhere to the east. The number of young dependants in the household had increased to seven siblings. Each day they faced the need for basic necessities of food and clothes. Survival was a daily challenge and living was hard for poor families on the island after the war years.

The short seasonal work to the American plantations that produced sugar cane, apples, banana and tobacco brought its financial rewards. This was readily apparent from those fortunate young men who secured the green card to travel. Such an opportunity was rear and had to be grabbed as though it was gold dust. The prospect of securing a Green Card for seasonal farm work in America would present some real problems for Ron. He may well have been all right on the requirement of the police record and on the physical fitness test. But he went to school only infrequently and could not be certain about the contents of his school record. He was unable to read or write and had a fear of needles so any prospect of an injection would be a hoop too far.

9

It was enviable to Ron and other young men with young dependant families that some of their peers were now leaving the island for seasonal work while the high rates of unemployment and the depression in domestic plantation farming continued. They all recognised that without the ability to earn money there would be very little chance to build the larger house necessary or buy even to buy a small plot of land for future security. A travelling party would consist of able-bodied young men who originated from various Caribbean and Latin American areas. Ships would collect the men at ports around the Caribbean before sailing to the farming states of Florida, Louisiana, Indiana and Maryland. Men shared basic communal facilities and secured living quarters for the duration of the season in which they harvested cotton, sugarcane, rice, fruits, tobacco, peanuts and other produce. As foreign labour workers they were granted the right of temporary entry to the States as part of a programme agreed between the Crown Colony Government and the receiving country. In the face of mass unemployment amongst the poorly educated and unskilled black population of the island, the outlet provided by seasonal plantation work was a source of relief. When the opportunity for seasonal work in America begun to fall away in the mid 1950s the growing number of unemployed unskilled labour on the island was tapped by the country that many generations had come to know as Great Britain: The Mother Country for the island colony.

Ron and his young family had now settled in Montpelier following the breakdown in relations between Lize and her sisters in Cascade during the period following the death of her father, Samuel Patterson. Montpelier would provide a fresh start and the prospect of living within a more supportive Riggan family circle. An opportunity was presented for Ron to join the band of young men who were touched by the tales that Great Britain offered easier access than America, with greater freedom to roam streets paved with gold. The choice most favoured by Ron and many of his peers was now quite straightforward.

It was generally agreed that the experience of farm labour was profitable and the seasonal climate largely favourable. The downside appeared to be the firm regime of racial segregation and physical isolation on large farms and plantations. The backdrop of violent civil rights struggles and the racial segregation against black people in America did not bode well with many prospective candidates from the island. But this reluctance was overcome when Ron saw family members leaving the island for seasonal work and would later return safely with earnings not previously thought possible. When the successful labour migrants showed the trappings of their new money in the purchase of land from absentee white landowners and then embarked upon building houses of wood and timber, the ambition of Lize and Ron became fully awakened. Ron gave due consideration to his options and came to a decision with his wife and young family. So instead of opting to sell his labour on the plantations of America, it was the choice of Great Britain that Ron would follow. The trip by boat from the island capital of Kingston was the first encounter he had with his new British passport, new grey suit and wide rimmed felt hat. Intervals of stopping and starting again at other island destination slowed the total journey time to nine weeks. It took a long time to see the shores of the Mother Country but they had finally arrived at the port of Southampton in late October 1957.

Chapter Two

Deep Roots

During the thirty years between 1957 and 1987 a pattern of chain migration would extend the branches of the family far beyond its island roots. A plan was agreed between Ron and Lize that would help to secure the future of their family. It fell upon him to leave the island and go to Britain to work for around five years. He would then come back home to his wife and young family where they could buy a piece of land and build a new house. The reality of their five years plan did not turn out as they expected. Ron had arrived in the industrial English Midland town of Walsall, near Birmingham. He had followed his brothers Cyril, Joslyn, Elijah, George and Moodie were already in Britain along with his sister Lillian. Ron and younger brother James arrived at the same time, with their youngest brother Lambert later completing the chain of migration within the primary family.

The company of physically fit young men with an eagerness to earn money may have served to give Ron a lapse into amnesia. He soon got into the British working culture of social drinking and late night partying and in a matter of eighteen months after arriving in the town he became a father for the eight time. At issue this time was the small matter that his wife was more than six thousand miles away in Jamaica. Lize was deeply wounded by the indiscretion of her husband. She felt that the man she trusted to fulfil his promise to their family had strayed. He had become somewhat foot loose and fancy free in Britain. He had betrayed his family. But Lize was not the kind of woman to sit by idly and watch her plan fall apart. She had her own contacts through the extended family network and they kept a close eye on Ron. The skill of wielding a mighty pen was put to good effect and the deep feeling of hurt in her heart was poured unto the page of each letter and would leave no doubt in Ron's head as to what their agreement was. It was not easy to ignore this woman when she believed herself to be swimming against an unkind current. She knew that her well-constructed plan was at serious risk of tumbling down and she needed to act fast. There was not time to think about the disgrace of losing her husband to an unknown world of public houses and women with whom she has never been acquainted.

Ron was aware that the money he had planned to earn for the land and new house had been steadily ebbed away by his newfound lifestyle. He didn't feel in a position to return without fulfilling the mission. There was also now the added complication that he had fathered a new child in Britain. Baby Thomas was born to an English mother in Walsall some three years after Ron had arrived in the area. Since he was an already married man with a dependant family and she was committed to be married to someone else, there was not much prospect of their bringing up their son happily together. Baby Thomas was adopted by an aunt and when Ron neglected his responsibility to provide financial support for the child, the matter of maintenance was put in the hands of the local magistrate court. He was not a literate man and for one with no previous history of having contact with the law in his own country, for this thing to happen in a foreign country it would have been very frightening. He had only just sent a letter in response to his wife to say he was not able to return home when her reply came back through the door:

Dear Mr Riggan,

I have just received your letter and see that you don't have the intention to return home to your children. Well let me tell you something, you could get one hundred pickney with English woman, I will stay here and put the law on you to make sure that you think say you too far to reach, mek me tell you, that would be a foolish mistake. You going to have to mind me and mind all seven children that you have here.

If you not going to come back home, then you tell me what is your plan? We don't have food to eat or clothes to wear. Is how you expect we to life? Is want you want me fe rob bank? Is prison you want to send me and send me children them on paupers roll? You damn out of order. We not good enough for you any more? mek me tell you something, a nearly twenty years me and you live. In all that time you never see or hear say me have another man. But you take up your self and gone with English woman.

Remember is who name Lize. Is me you married to. Me name wife and is me send you go a Britain. And me not going to stand by and watch you follow rum bar and English woman and bring disgrace upon me family. You better get on the next ship and come home or your corner going to be dark. Remember say me Lize tell you so.

15

Your Wife,
Mrs Lize Riggan

Many other letters followed from the smoking pen wielded by Lize over the next months. There was really no way to find a reprieve for Ron. That is until a further letter from his wife completely turns the tables. Instead of the angry demands that he return home, she suggested this time that he should pay the air ticket for her and the three oldest children to bring them to Britain instead. The plan did not have much appeal to Ron and he let his wife know that he was unable to meet the cost of their travel. The impatience peaked with the slow pace of reply coming back from Ron was further exacerbated by having to cope alone with the growing pains of their teenage children at home. She was especially concerned for the immediate future of the fast maturing older girls, Bibs and Earva.

When the funds from Ron slowed to merely a solitary drip at Christmas, Easter and August, Lize promptly secured the support of her sister-in-law Lillian, who was already in England, and borrowed the money needed to meet the cost of travel for their eldest daughter. The dispatch of the sixteen year old Bibs from the island was intended as the first step before all three older children could be settled with their father. They could each find work and make a contribution to the cost of travel for Lize and the remaining siblings. But it turned out that only Bibs made it to England in 1960 as the plan quickly disintegrated following the shotgun courtship and marriage by the teenager. This latest sway from the plan set in place by Lize was almost too much for her to take and in a matter of a few months she had arrival at Ron's door at 22 Milton Street in Walsall. It wasn't long before there was a new wind of change in Ron's behaviour. The visits to the public house became much less frequent and now occurred only at weekends. Accounting for the fortnightly earning was now the preserve of his wife. The intention was clear. The cat was back and the mice had to disappear from view at least. Lize recognised that the earning power of a single breadwinner was rather limiting her ambition to bring the remaining six children to Britain from Jamaica. She therefore went out to work at a nearby clothing factory and where she was again presented with the opportunity to exercise the skill of dress making and sewing. Two breadwinners meant the independence of a rented house and the control over the outflow of their earnings. That is, until there was further pita patter of two little feet; then there were four and them six sets of tiny feet as addition to the family overseas. Teenage bride Bibs added the first pita, then with almost precision timing, both mother and daughter delivered new baby boys in the same maternity ward at the Walsall Manor Hospital in the heart of winter, December 1962. There is a real cost to be put against child rearing in Britain and while being outwardly delighted in the health and joy of their fifth son, Lize knew deep down in her heart that the steering wheels had again been wrenched away from the intended course. She started to wonder to herself, "Is it my faith that I am going to be separated from the rest of my children?"

The tears could not be helped as she prayed in the darkened room of the maternity ward the night following the natural birth of the child at just two minutes into Boxing Day.

> *"Lord, I know you is God and you can make a way for me to see all my children again. Lord a thank you for the blessing of baby Jimmy, but Lord, me a beg you to let me find a way to take up all of me other children. You know that them need me, Lord. Me need them too. And Lord, help me children them in Jamaica so that they*

have something to eat for Christmas. I'm not there to look after them and Lord, me asking you to protect them."

She hardly noticed the gale of the snowstorm against the single glazed window of the maternity ward. The midwife had arrived to perform her after birth routine. It was snowing outside but the pain and soreness from her hardest labour was temporarily forgotten as her mind drift slowly across the Atlantic to her children who were still on the island.

Chapter Three

Foreign Branches

Four months had passed slowly when the worst winter on record gave way to a peep of blue sky behind high grey clouds. Baby Jimmy looked alert and some older family members volunteered to baby-sit if Lize wanted to go back to work. Conscious of the pressure being absorbed by the pocket of her husband, she had thought about matters and took the opportunity to take another job since the foreman of the previous sewing factory had expressed his displeasure at the expecting forty year old. This was a disruption to the business and he would not be taking her on again.

By the arrival of Christmas of the following year the level of concern over the separation of the family was again brought to the forefront of her mind. They had managed to save enough money to meet the cost of travel for the next two older children. Ken was now eighteen, Earva was sixteen and Vandley fourteen years old. They were living in the care of grandmother Estry in Montpelier. The old lady was advancing in years and the reports reaching Lize caused her real concerns. She had read from one letter that," Miss Estry can't manage your children.

Sometimes she is leaving them at home by themselves while she goes out to sport and enjoy herself."

The relationship between Lize and her mother, Estry, was at best distant and was in part due to a feeling of rejection by the illegitimate daughter who felt that her very conception and birth was the source of embarrassment. Estry was married at the time with a separate family when the child was conceived with Samuel Patterson of Cascade. The already established family never accepted the young Lize and the rejection was complete when at age four she was rescued by her married father. He had at least made a sacrifice of separating from his wife and taking in the child.

By force of circumstance, Lize felt quite obligated to use one hand to wash the other. At a distance of more than six thousand miles, each had a need for the other. Estry was asked to move to the house vacated by Lize and care for the six remaining children. Funds for maintaining the children and the upkeep of food and clothes would be provided by Lize. It was never going to be a contract of trust and almost from the start some strong suspicion had aroused in her heart and head. It troubled her that Estry had not proved herself to be a good mother and it troubled her that Estry had more of a reputation for being sporting and spendthrift. There was a niggling suspicion that at least part of the funds sent for the care of her six children would be consumed on the dependent children of the sisters and brothers who had rejected her. She was not yet ready to forgive them. She remembered that they had hurried her departure from her home in the district of Cascade a decade earlier. She was already asking herself the question as she drifted into another night of interrupted sleep with a teething baby.

"Why should me stay here and send Estry me hard earned money to spend on herself and man?"

She thought further, "Them kids said they never get the things that I sure send in that parcel for them. If them don't get it, then who is getting them? Well I think Estry is giving away me things to other people and them children."

The heart was heavy and troubled and Lize continued to lament in the presence of Ron.

"Lord God, please, me begging you, don't let Estry take advantage of me and me children. You know that I am not there to see to it that they will get the things I buy and send over for them. And God, a pray that you will make Estry stop take things away from my children."

The tears were never far away and it was getting to Ron. His wife always seemed to have her mind in another world although the body was present with him.

"Lize, why don't you stop the worry about it? You can't do anything about it if your mother is using out the money we send?"

He expected her to react.

"Me can do something about it. And let me tell you something else, is fe me pickney them and me not going to stand here and watch Estry take advantage of them."

"What you can do about it then?" protested Ron.

"Not a thing!" was the reply.

Lize continued in earnest seriousness, "You can stay right here and worry about rum bottle and other woman, but me a go take care of me pickney them."

When another letter arrived to inform her that her second daughter Earva was keeping bad company and going to dance with boys the rest of the world may well have stood still. The swirl of confusion and frustration floating in Lize's head was beyond her powers of containment. The water in the saucepan on top of the small cooker in the corner of the kitchen had long evaporated and was now starting to burn on the heat. She heard the turn of Ron's key in the front door and the next few seconds she again heard the anxiety of his raised voice in the kitchen.

"Lize, you burning down the house! You don't see you set fire to the pan on the fire?"

"What fire?" asked a startled Lize, entering the same side of the kitchen. Ron gestured intently with both hands, "You a burn up the pan on the stove!"

Her eyes trailed to the corner of the kitchen.

"Tun off the stove! Tun it off and get some water!" Her mood had quickly become one of panic.

The fire was put out and the only damage was the blackened saucepan and the smoke filled kitchen. That scare of a full-scaled fire would pass but the source of Lize's anxiety was far from abated. There were just too many tales reaching her to lament the children's drift out of control and the exposure of the teenagers to the influences of the music and rebellion of the swinging sixties. The craze of the fashionable mini skirt was already a big hit with Earva and she would wear the garment and the name for many years. If ever there was a straw which broke the back of the camel, then it came shortly afterwards when the travel fare was finally raised and sent to Estry for the booking to be made and the children dispatched to England. The reply that came back to Lize was not the one she had anticipated at all.

The Sunday was spent in church and Lize felt justified in raising her hands skyward and ringing wholehearted praise in the name of God. Surely it was by the grace and mercy of the Saviour above in the heaven that had made it possible for them to save the money that was now in the hands of

Estry. She would be trusted to go ahead as instructed by the accompanying letter to ask the Justice of the Peace in the neighbouring town of Sandy Bay, Hanover, to sign the passport forms for the two youngest children and then get their travel ticket to Southampton. It was almost Easter and if she really get moving the children would arrive by the end of summer. The same instructions were conveyed to Ken as the oldest of the remaining six children on the island. Ken didn't need much time to consider the instructions. After all he had received them before and had his own passport ready at hand when Bibs went by herself. The same passport was at hand when Lize left them with the promise that it wouldn't be long and she would be sending for all of them. The period of almost three years had passed quite quickly for Ken. No longer the strong bruising boy of fifteen, he had completed school and was now actively involved in the life of the local New Testament Church of God in Montpelier. The grown ups often said he was a natural leader of his peers and one day they expected him to become a great leader of the church. He knew deep down that he would much prefer to remain in the church and with the group of friends who he knew well. There was an opportunity to take up training at the main Bible College to the east of the island and this was now the main preoccupation of the young man.

Lize had always known that her oldest son had a stubbornness that could be unbreakable when tested. But somehow she expected him to respond favourably to her request that he should travel to England to join her. The passage from the letter received from Estry had to be read over and over again.

"The boy say him don't want to come to England. Him want fe go turn church Minister. Him say he going to study Bible in one place up the line name St Mary. I don't even know where that place is. Some people tell me say that is where Church of God people them go learn to turn Minister. The boy must want to turn Minister, else him would never gone."

The remaining text in the letter might well have disappeared from the page as Lize read the letter. She had cried before and prayed to God but somehow, this was a different kind of crying. She felt the numbing of her body and spirit in a moment that felt like an age. A pen and paper was already in her hand when she sat at the table and started to write. She stopped to wipe the stream of tears from both cheeks. The crackling of her voice was desperately held deep and suppressed in her belly. More tears streamed down under the rim of the dark framed glasses. The soul was tormented. The head was giddy. Her thoughts came out with the striking of the tightly clinched left fist.

"How can the boy do this after all the try me try?" More tears streamed down the face.

" Me have to get somebody who can go talk sense in his head." Another attempt is made to focus the eyes and the pen to the writing pad. The latest sheet of screwed up paper sailed across the room. The only words she was able to get down on the piece of paper followed the implosion of her deep anger. She started,

> Dear Pastor Curniffe,
> I am begging you to talk to Ken and let him see sense. Please talk to him and tell him say

The flow of thought was much too consuming and confused to complete any of the several attempts made to construct a new letter. The build up of anxiety exploded into a further sea of tears because she was deeply troubled by her family.

Baby Jimmy was sleeping comfortably in the middle of the bed in the room. Ron was doing day shift at work and Bibs was living a few miles away with her husband, Clive Stewart, and two children, Melva aged three and Floyd a year younger and a similar age to his uncle Jimmy. The family she was so desperate to reconstruct had just been shattered into a pile of irretrievable pieces and Lize felt deep in the gut that this time the break up was fatal. The letters were written eventually over the following days. The theme was the same. Some of the words she employed were exact.

"Please talk to the boy and show him sense. Him don't realise what he is saying. I already send the money to Estry to buy the travel tickets for all of them. Please talk to the boy for me, and show him sense."

The minister of the local church replied first. Other replies followed from the Justice of the Peace and also from the postmistress, the retired head teacher and the local elected Councillor. The two oldest uncles and the two oldest aunts also replied to their letters. When each was read five or six times the tear ducts were near empty. Each letter made her cry more than the last. The period of six or eight days between their arrival did not help the anticipation of further emotional anguish. The one line seemed to be present over and over again:

"Lize, I talk to Ken but him say his mind is made up. He doesn't want to go to Britain. He wants to go to Bible College. He want to be a minister in the church."

It was a feeling of de ja vu. Each letter repeated the same words. They were written over and over again on each page. Ron wished he could do something to fix the situation for his wife but knew that short of springing a miracle and bringing all six children from Jamaica to Britain, he could be of no assistance. He prepared food to the cry of mother and child. He knew that this was not for the first time and was not likely to be for the last. When his eyes fell on the face of his wife from across the vacant space between kitchen and bedroom, he felt deeply sore and uncertain of what else could be done. But her name was Lize. There is something else that she will be able to do.

The days and nights rolled by without any real distinction. Both were darkened by the clouds hovering in the early autumn sky and by the tired tear filled eyes. Hundreds of thoughts had already gone through her head and each linked to a turn around in the situation and bringing the six children to Britain. Ken had not yet replied to the last two letters from his mother. Maybe he was thinking about things again. Important people had spoken to him and he had seen sense. Lize was up from her bed before the postman reached the door again. It had been the same level of anticipation for eight weeks at least. The whistling postman knew her by first name and by voice. He was uttering some usually friendly words to her, "You have any letter for me today?" Her eyes remained fixed to the sagging weight in blue canvas bag being carried over the shoulders.

"Oh yes, Lize, I always has something for you!"

The broad smile on the face of the postman disguised the cutting chill of the cold morning air. The postman may have handed her four or five items but the only thing she noticed in the moment was the red and blue edged letters stamped "Airmail". One was from Ken. Lize hurried the fingers under the edge to break the seal without disturbing the carefully folded paper content. She surveyed each word on each line while the pendulum of her head shift from left to right. The heart was pounding faster. She was trying to read too quickly and one or two words may have been missed. She sat down and read the letter from her son again.

Dear *Mother,*
I have received your two letters. I see what you have to say, but I not going to bother to come to Britain. I already apply to go to Bible College and they said I can start next month. I already have somewhere to live and I don't want to come over to Britain. I want to stay here and work for the church as a minister. Pastor Curniffe said he will help me and some of the church brothers and church sisters said they will help me if me need anything.

The money that you send for the travel for all of us can still pay for Earva, Roxy, Denzil, Noreen and Barry. All of them could still come if they want but Earva said she don't want to come. The others them said they don't want to come to Britain either. So nobody don't want to come over there. Them say that them wa' to stay here.

Me could take some of the money to pay for me College and Estry can have the rest to buy food and clothes for them other children. But me don't want to come over there again and the others don't want to come over there either. Me don't know if you will write to me again but me don't want to come over there. I will prefer to stay here and study and serve God.

Your son,
Ken

Chapter Four

New Shoots

The doctor meant well with his advice that Lize would put herself and the unborn child at risk if she insisted on travelling more than six thousand miles on a passenger ship from Southampton to Kingston in Jamaica. She had more than enough time to think about this and her mind was fully made up. Both Ron and Bibs tried to persuade her to delay travelling until after the child was born in the New Year. Since Ken did not want to come to Britain and Earva was not straying from home and from the control of her grandmother Estry, there was no real alternative but to pay her own passage and go home to her six children. Brother-in-law Moodie and his wife was already booked to travel to Jamaica from Southampton in two weeks time and Lize was determined to be on the ship with them.

"You shouldn't travel with that big belly", Ron tried to insist but to no avail.

"What else you want me to do, eh? You want me to sit down here when me pickney them a go astray?" The eyes were serious and resigned.

"But you nearly seven months pregnant, and the doctor already say you shouldn't travel. It too dangerous and the weather soon turn bad."

Lize knew deep in her heart that everyone who bothered to give her advice to her face and warned her about the danger to herself and the unborn child was right. But she just didn't feel that the situation could be helped. In her mind she went through the full range of thoughts about the risks and dangers of travelling. There was the concern about the Earva. Ken had informed her in the latest letter that Earva was not behaving herself and that when he tried to exercise discipline she went away from the house with some friends and said she was not coming back home. He had tried to forcefully return her to the family home but she had been adamant on leaving. There was nothing else he could have done about his younger sister. Since he was not settled in at Bible College more than one hundred miles away to the east of the island, there were only four children left in the care of grandmother Estry.

Lize had written ahead nearly five weeks before to instruct Estry to use the money available for the travel to purchase three acres of land that had come up for sale in the district. She thought that at least something good had come from the debacle to her family caused by Ken. That piece of land had now been secured and she intended to build a new wooden house on it. Estry had also been instructed to ask the best carpenter in the district to make a start on raising up the building. It was hoped that one or two rooms could be completed by the time she docked in Kingston at the end of November.

"Ron, why you don't let the two of us go home with Moodie and his wife?".

"How me and you to go home now? What me to go home to do?". He had become resigned to a further fate of his wife leaving without him. But he felt it was not good sense for her to even be thinking of travelling in the state of pregnancy. It was even worse to think about going home without enough money. Ron had also been thinking about the options for the past few weeks. The constant worry in his head made him increase the visits to the public house. All his family and friends agreed with his view that Lize was being foolish about travelling back to Jamaica when she was heavily pregnant. She was nearly forty-two years old. In Ron's mind the whole thing was mad.

At last the day of travel to Southampton had arrived. Moodie and his wife Lillian were ready with their children. Bibs had persuaded her mother to take her two children to Jamaica as well ahead of her return with Clive. They travelled together on a coach from Walsall to Southampton. The dock seemed overcrowded with passenger ships, ferries, luxury liners and private cruise boats. The travel tickets bore the ship's name "The Big Horn". During the next forty days or so that vessel became their home. Ron was alone again as the swinging door was closed behind each passenger as they filed through port control. Brother in law Moodie filled the role as substitute for his brother Ron who stood and waved his wife and child and grand children goodbye. He was sorry to see them go and the quite unconscious frown remained with the first darkened lines that had appeared during the past months. His body was starting to feel the wear and strains of his forty-two years and how he reflected back on the only other time in October 1957 when he travelled on a coach between this very port and the industrial town of Walsall. The excitement of going into the unknown was not present now. It felt like he had been here before but hoped that he hadn't and that he would be returning home to his wife and baby Jimmy. But of course that would be the case and he was alone again with no way of knowing how long this would continue to be the case. Ron's eyes closed as his body again adjusted to the jerking and rocking of the coach. He hoped his wife would arrive on the island safely.

The living and sleeping quarters of the ship felt like it was buried deep in the belly of the large vessel. Six weeks felt like a never-ending age. There had been five or six occasions to visit the medical centre so far but there had not really been any alarm. Checking the blood pressure and heart beat were the normal concerns for expecting mothers at an advanced state of their pregnancy. Lize was now over twenty-nine weeks and she could not be certain that she would make it to land before her water would break. She was feeling tired more easily and was permitted to receive all her main meals in her sleeping quarter. She felt a strong urge to push the baby out.

"Doctor, a going to start!"

She was visibly anxious and he tried to reassure her.

"You are not due quite as yet, Mrs Riggan. But you must try to rest and stay calm for me."

"But doctor, how you can expect me to stay calm when we moving on water day and night?"

"You will feel somewhat anxious by the motion of the vessel, from time to time. But I have examined you and baby will not be coming out for a few weeks yet."

She was not convinced.

"A can feel everything moving you know doctor. And a starting to feel like pushing."

The grey haired medic placed a reassuring hand on Lize's shoulder. "You must stop worrying, Mrs Riggan. Because if you do, we will be forced to get baby out early."

"A don't want to have this baby on the ship, you know doctor. A don't want to have no sea baby." After a brief pause, she asked, "And a what nationality the baby will have if him born on the ship, sir?"

The doctor smiled. "The baby will be fine and you will be alright too. We are here to take the best care of you and baby."

Brother-in-law Moodie and his wife were always helpful during the trip and they kept a sharp eye out for the children as they scampered about on all levels and decks. Baby Jimmy had caught the eyes of a Spanish couple on board. The man seemed especially keen to offer the child sweets. When he asked Lize whether she would mind if he and his wife could take the child on a walk on deck she said she didn't mind as long as he undertook to bring the child back safely. Sergio and his wife Maria took a strong liking to the toddler and as they were about to depart at their destination in the Dominica Republic they approached Lize and asked whether she would consider letting them take Jimmy. She could quite understand what they were asking, but she believed they were asking to take the child permanently and giving her some sort of payment.

"No sah, that is my child and he is not for sale." Lize felt her blood pressure raising as she secured her son and two grandchildren and waddled away down the steps towards her sleeping quarter.

"What you think him is, a slave?" The anger was tangible.

Lize continued to remonstrate, "Mi son is not for sale." She fixed a stern gaze on Maria's face. Although she spoke very little English that look in her eyes translated very clearly in Spanish and any other language that Maria had cared to speak.

"This is my baby. Not yours. And him is not for sale to you or to anybody else in this world."

She could again feel the stress of the situation moving through her body. The doctor had advised her to stay calm. She didn't want to go into a premature labour and would not be taking any further chance with anyone else during the final twenty-four hours of the journey.

The skies were dark with a constellation of bright stars arranged at intervals of roughly the same distance between each one. The passengers could now disembark from The Big Horn at the port in Kingston. The time was almost 10:30 p.m. but judging by the size of the milling crowd Lize could be forgiven for thinking that the entire population of the capital were assembled at the port. Moodie helped to collect the women and children from their interrupted sleep. He navigated them to the waiting area at the port and when they were all seated had again set off this time to the luggage bay. He already knew that only the smaller pieces of their luggage would be received and the port authority would dispatch the heavier items that he and Ron had sent by freight during the following fourteen days. Moodie spotted a dark leather grip on which that his wife had written the name and address: "*Stanley Riggan, Cascade PA, Hanover, Jamaica, West Indies.*" He would wait to collect each of the seven remaining cases and also the five that belonged to Lize. The waiting seemed to have taken forever when the last grip was collected. Moodie secured a large luggage trolley from a port assistant and begun his march through the exit door beyond which his wife waited to guard the items while he returned for a further trip. The travelling party were soon reassembled together with their luggage. They would now follow the flow of the crowd to go out into the Kingston night and the waiting relatives and friends massed to meet and greet the returnees.

Ken was among the waiting relatives. His heart was filled with anticipation of seeing his mother again after more than four years. He was also aware of the letters they had exchanged and her words urging him to change his mind and come to Britain with the other children. They had disagreed on that issue but tonight he would only be interested in seeing her safe return. Ken took up a position close to the front of the waiting crowd. He wanted to see his mother as soon as she appeared through the exit gate. As the wait continued he wondered whether she would look the same way as he remembered from the time that she left the island. She had since given birth to a new baby in Britain. Ken imagined that his baby brother would be walking by now since he was nearly two years old. He thought further about whom the boy looked like? His fleeting thoughts went first to the facial features of Ron, or maybe even like Barry. He couldn't be certain, but it didn't really matter in that moment just whom the boy looked like. He was born in Britain, so maybe the little boy would be white!

"See her there!", Amos shouted, thinking that he had spotted Lize before his friend did.

"No man", Ken reacted, "Is not her that".

Amos responded again, "Is she, yes"

"Is not Lize that. I say you wrong again".

Ken was even more certain that his friend was wrong when the woman picked out by his friend Amos passed them close by. She was tall and brown in complexion. Ken thought that the woman did look a little bit like Lize though.

"See your uncle Moodie coming there"

Amos was right this time and the smile on the man's face was unmistakable.

"Uncle Moodie, uncle Moodie"

Ken motioned with both arms raised above his head and caught the attention of his uncle. The meeting party all collected around Moodie with information about the waiting truck and questions about the other family members. Moodie pointed in the direction of the waiting women and children. The meeting party went on ahead and quickly put into motion the transfer of luggage from the port building to the waiting truck. Ken was walking more slowly than the others when his eyes fell upon the face of his mother. He wanted to move more quickly to embrace her. But he could not propel his legs to move forward. His only conscious thought was wrapped up with his gaze on

34

the large stomach being carried by Lize. The shock to his wide-open eyes was for the unexpected state of pregnancy but in the falling of Ken's jaws there was the horror that the baby in his mother's protruding stomach was just about ready to pop out! On the side of the harbour! Tonight! Lize could just about waddle forward under the weight of her ninth pregnancy.

The two women in the travelling party went to take up the seats at the front of the vehicle near the driver. Moodie and the other children went to take to the back of the truck under the area covered by tarpaulin. The journey to Hanover would take around four hours. They were all aboard with their luggage and leaving the lights of Kingston Harbour behind them. The flurry of earlier conversations had thinned out after the half waypoint through the journey home. A thick pane of glass behind the driver created a rear windscreen between the passengers. There was a single hanging light bulb hanging from a piece of string under the tarpaulin. The truck rocked to a slow pedestrian pace in order to avoid the large hole in the middle of the road. The bright headlight beamed ahead in the distance as the amplified sound of the gear changing quickly from first to second and then to third. Rocking and seemingly stumbling around deep and curving corners and close to the edge of open gullies and falls, the driver continued the journey westward along the main A1 route of the island's north coast.
"Is where we reach now?", asked Amos.
The question was not aimed at anyone in particular, just perhaps to those still awake through the journey.
"We soon reach Discovery Bay", Twidley replied.
"And about how much more miles 'till Falmouth?"
Twidley was not sure but he felt the need to provide the younger enquirer with an answer.

"After Discovery Bay we 'av to reach one place name Duncans, and after that is when we a go reach Falmouth".

Amos seemed content with the information provided by Twidley about the areas and distance that was still to be travelled before they reached home. Ken was still awake and eaves dropping on the information. The trailing road left behind by the vehicle was still black in the darkness of the moonless sky. He could not see any clear body form through the thick rear screen of the truck but assumed that Lize and Lillian sitting beside her would be fast asleep. Uncle Moodie was certainly sleeping and the rhythm of the loud snoring bears testimony to that fact. The children slouching next to him were all comfortably sleeping as the truck shook to changing of the gears before labouring around a deep bend to the right and then to the left of the narrow asphalt road. They passed the bright street lights in the well kept grounds of the Great House in Rose Hall. Hanover would follow the Parish of St James and they knew that after four hours their journey would soon come to its end.

Hopewell was quiet at 3 a.m. in the morning with only the overhead streetlights positioned above the shopping area. The chorus of cock-a-doodle-do by roosters in the passing yards seemed the only thing that was alert to the heavy rolling engine of the truck. Amos peeped through the dark of the emerging morning to the landmark information painted onto the side of a light coloured wall: "1 Mile Sandy Bay".

"We reach now!", he alerted his friend Ken.

They attempted to peel away the closed tarpaulin at the back of the truck to reveal the breaking of a new day. The vehicle turned left next to the sign clearly marked "Sandy Bay Police Station". It would now travel the short distance of just over one and a half miles up the hilly and uneven single tracked road going in a southbound direction from the coastal town of Sandy Bay to the heavily wooded district of Montpelier.

When the journey was completed Lize felt a keen sense of disorientation. The environment that she had previously known and retained in her memory had changed. Almost nothing was recognisable in her first moments after being helped from the front seat of the truck. Luggage of grips and trunks, bags and boxes that carried the written label "*Sybil E. Riggan, Montpelier District, Sandy Pay PO, Hanover, Jamaica, West Indies*", were taken from amongst the cargo shared between the two families of Lize and Moodie. The welcome party of boys and men all assisted to collect and transport the items by their heads, hands, back and by doubling up to carry the load to the safety of the semi-completed family home. Soon the truck would go back down the hill to Sandy Bay before making its journey westward to Cascade district with Moodie and his family.

"Mim reach home!" The sound of her children's voices was unfamiliar to Lize. She attempted to identify each one as they emerged from the house to meet their mother. The youngest of the children she had left on the island was Barry. He had not long passed his eighth birthday. Noreen was just two years older than her brother, while Denzil was just about to enter his teenage years. At fifteen, Vandley was the next oldest child behind the seventeen-year-old Earva. Ken was her senior by a further two years. Their new brother Jimmy was introduced to all of them and the toddler seemed to be bursting with a new surge of excitement as he attempted to survey all the rooms in the house. They were introduced to their first niece Melva, and nephew, Floyd. Lize had already noted that another of her children was missing. She looked across at Ken. He turned his face away from her gaze because both their thoughts were as one at that moment. Earva was missing somewhere on the island and Lize wanted her at home with the family.

Chapter Five

Lost and Found

By the outbreak of day all the visible signs of the truck had passed and the sound of local voices crept into the space around the slightly opened window in the bedroom occupied by Lize. Her eyes and ears would need more time to readjust to the vacuous sounds of barking dogs, mooing of cows and the squealing of domestic pigs. The heavy mix of sounds merged into a unique rhythm of life on the island that she had almost forgotten. She yielded from the temptation to remain in her state of slumber. The heavy stomach was now settled after a few hours of discomfort. She raised her body to a position where she was able to peep quietly through a gap in the glass window.

The scene of green grass and flowers bathing in the morning sun was a welcome change to the damp and grey sky of the English Midlands. The physical space around the room she now occupied was open and marked by an absence of locked doors. There was no carriageway in front of the house with the hazard of speeding cars outside to which she had become accustomed in Britain. Here there were no signs of factories with their clattering press of metal, iron and steel and industrial machinery. There was no bellowing of black stained smoke through domestic and industrial chimneys. She would have no need for coal fire and paraffin heaters. The atmospheric air of the island was warm and clean with a gentle rustling of sea breeze against sheets of zinc arranged on the roof of wooden houses.

Estry did not raise from her sleep in the early hours as the grandchildren in her care rushed from their adjoining bedrooms to greet their mother. She had thought about getting up to extend her own greeting to her youngest daughter but had hesitated and the opportune moment seemed to have passed. Her reticence was due in no short measure to the strong defence she had offered in her final letter in response to her daughter's claim that the children left in her care were going astray. That accusation was taken by Estry as confirmation that her daughter was suspicious of her ability to care for her grandchildren. Estry didn't feel that she needed to demonstrate any further proof to her own daughter. She had harboured the thought in her head that if Lize thought herself to be a better parent than she was, then maybe it was right that she should return from Britain to care for her own children. She did not feel herself to be any more responsible for the decision taken by Ken to defy the wish of his mother and opt to stay on the island rather than travel to England. Neither did she feel that it was due to any neglect on her part as to why Earva had left home and the district with her friends to live in the island's second city of Montego Bay.

The twenty four-foot length of the veranda separated mother and daughter. Their eyes collided. Each walked into the same vacant space towards each other. Estry broke the silence.

"Hello Lize", she walked towards her daughter with a half smile on her face. Her eyes concealed her expectation of a hostile response from her daughter. The grey shoulder length hair was uncovered. The pale complexion of the face was served by a flush of adrenaline around the body.

"Mornin' Miss Estry", came the brief response from Lize. The walk slowed to a halt under the weight of her heavily pregnant stomach. The hands of the two women didn't touch but they stood close enough to be able to hear any word whispered from one to the other.

"Me glad fe see you arrive safely", Estry continued.

"And the children them really glad too." She did not draw the response expected from her daughter.

"Me did hear the truck when it reach last night but me didn't want to get in the way and me know say you woulda tired to."

Lize continued to look in the general direction of her mother's face but was conscious not to convey the pent-up hostility that was being held back inside.

"Yes, we arrive safe with Moodie and Lillian. They should reach home to Cascade long time now."

Jimmy came over to join his mother and grandmother in their tepid conversation.

"This is me son." Lize motioned to the child.

Estry observed her daughter in the strained posture of a heavily pregnant woman.

"And mi see say you will give us another one very soon."

She turned her gaze from her daughter's stomach to acknowledge the toddler and confirmed that Noreen had already introduced her to her grandson earlier in the morning.

"Dog! The toddler pointed to the small black and while puppy sitting down on the steps of the house.

"My dog?" he asked.

Floyd and Melva joined their uncle Jimmy on the veranda of the house as the older children petted the new arrivals from Britain.

"You like de puppy?" Estry asked the child.

"Dog! Bite!" Jimmy said in response to his grandmother.

"No, him naa go bite you."

Estry looked down into the innocent eyes of the boy.

Melva sought further reassurance.

"Grandma, will dog bite if I hold it?"

Estry raised her eyes to notice that Lize had returned from the veranda to the adjoining bedroom. The door remained open and she was already in the process of unpacking some of the grips and bags. Her advanced pregnancy gave the upright posture a look of a sagging package amongst the luggage. Estry continued to give her attention to the children gathered near her feet. She provided her great granddaughter with a response of further reassurance. She reached down to the puppy with her right hand and patted the head and neck. The children followed her to touch the puppy and compete for its attention. Estry was now conscious that some further time would be necessary to overcome the distance that had become apparent in her daughter. She watched briefly as Lize gave her attention to the luggage heaped together on the floor of the bedroom. She was able to sort the main items that each contained. Some bags contained items of clothing and footwear brought for each of her children. There were new dresses brought for Estry and trousers for her nephew Twidley. Other bags contained tinned food, beans, peanuts, sweets, oils, bottles of tonic wine and other items she had brought before she left Britain some six weeks ago. In time she would share these out and everyone would receive their bounty from England.

When Ken came into his mother's room he again surveyed the stacks of leather grips and cases that they had removed from the truck. He had not quite realised the large quantity of the cargo. They seemed to have filled the entire floor space in two large adjacent rooms, in addition to taking up most of the standing room available in the bedroom.

"Mim, you want anything?" he asked Lize.

"No, not right now, but a want you to go and find Earva and tell her say me call her".

Ken had anticipated this request and had already sent word to inform his sister that their mother had arrived home safely. He felt bound to encourage Earva to return home for even a brief visit. In his mind he was prepared to wait until later in the week to see whether his sister would put in an appearance. If that failed, then he would bring into action a contingency plan to go direct to the address of the room in Montego Bay. Ken had written the name of the street given for Earva and her friends in Montego Bay, but he suddenly had a renewed sense of uncertainty. He didn't recognise the name of the street that was written on the piece of brown coloured paper. His enquiry from people in the district who he knew to be frequent visitors to the markets in Mo-Bay did not provide him with the certainty that he was seeking about the location of the address. When Lize again raised the question with him, he felt some trepidation from his uncertainty about the exact address and whether his sister would still be residing there.

"I not gonna wait another day to see me pickney".

Lize's voice invaded the quiet void in the room. Ken recognised the resoluteness in his mother's voice. He knew that she meant every word she had just uttered.

"Me want her home. This is where she should be. She is only a pickney."

The mode of speech was a mix of Jamaican Creole and the sounds of English words acquired from the limited communication Lize had with native English work mates, the

42

mailman, shopkeepers and Saturday market traders during the four years of living in Britain.

"I don't understand why she leave home in the first place?"

Lize was conscious that Estry was present in the close proximity of a room at the back of the house. Her mother was not physically visible but she had reckoned on her mother being within earshot of every word spoken.

Lize continued to measure her words although not intending to direct them at any named individual.

"After me give clear instructions to book the passage for all me pickney them. I send enough money what me labour to earn inna cold factory in Britain. And what happen to it?"

The pause was quite deliberate. Ken's discomfort was growing and he recognised that his mother's words were aimed at not only Estry but at himself also. He recognised that the question posed was rhetorical. He didn't need to offer an answer. He coiled his body across the bed with his face down on his folded arms as Lize continued her quarrel.

"Just to book the passage. That was all what I asked people to do for me pickney them."

The grievance was very clear if not her antagonist.

"Just fe book the passage and pay the money that me send. But even that was too much to ask people to do."

The volume in the voice was increasing. Ken knew that the comment was aimed at him, at least in part.

"The same God that them serve here is the same God in Britain."

The raw emotion and hurt in the voice was not disguised.

"I don't see why oonu couldn't all come to Britain. Oonu woulda find more opportunity and find good work. Oonu coulda buy house and car if oonu want. Nobody would stop oonu."

Ken remained silent. He knew his mother had been very badly hurt by his decision to renege on the promise to take his place behind his elder sister Bibs and travel to Britiain to join her and Ron. He knew that his decision to stay on the island had effectively forced Lize to return so abruptly to the island. Lize and Ron had become separated by his decision, at least temporarily, and he was very conscious of that fact. He recognised that Earva had left home during the period of uncertainty as letters passed between Lize, Estry and himself. She had taken exception to his attempt to move into the role as head of the family in the absence of their parents and the casual laissez faire approach to guardianship adopted by Estry.

"Before day light tomorrow, we going to find me pickney and carry her home."

Ken accepted the challenge lay down by his mother. He didn't need to speak any word on the matter. He stood up from the bed and collected his shoe from the veranda. During the next hours he would try to arrange for a taxi to take them on the thirty-five miles round trip to the city of Montego Bay in the neighbouring parish of St James.

The car journey to Montego Bay didn't appear to take as long as Lize was anticipating. The bumps and ridges on some tracks of road made for some discomfort in her advanced state of pregnancy. But the matter of distance and the build up of the mid-morning humidity was not the main source of worry in her mind. The hired car came to a stop at a street that Ken hoped was the residence of his sister. He was surprised at the speed of movement generated by his mother as she hastily alight from the car. The heavy stomach did not impede her steps. Already she was in the full flow of a wobbling walk. She was ahead of Ken and venturing to enter the open gateway to the tenement building at the address written on the piece of paper in their possession. Lize didn't notice any of the passers-by that had now turned to gaze in her direction. A slender chain restricted the movement of a dog that was present in the yard. It was barking quite rapturously but none of this could divert from the source of her attention.

A young woman emerged on the veranda at the front of the tenement house. She stood to look at the heavily pregnant stranger who was clearly heading in her direction. From the ever-reducing distance between them Lize looked at her for not more than a brief moment and continued her approach to the side of the house where a second entrance was visible. Ken pointed to the entry as the room occupied by his sister. The door to the room was open and a young woman was visible from inside. Lize thought that the young woman was perhaps slightly older than she had expected Earva to be. The young woman did not appear to have noticed Lize even as she got closer to the doorway. Lize kept her eyes on the young woman. She emerged up the three steps to the side of the building to stand in her sagging posture before the door of the room.

"Where is Earva?" questioned Lize.

Startled by the expression of serious intent by the heavily pregnant stranger, the young woman's response may have been delayed for only a few seconds, although Lize was quite impatient for a reply when the next question was released.

"I said where is me daughter? She don't live here with you?"

A quizzical brow was raised on the face of the young woman before she responded.

"But I don't know who you looking for, lady?"

"No. She don't live at this house anymore".

The young woman was visibly startled by the intensity of the moment. She was not familiar with the face of her inquisitor but succumbed to her suspicion that the woman standing there was the mother of her former roommate.

"So where she is? Where she moved gone? You don't know?"

The look of serious intent on Lize's face was clear.

"How you mean you don't know. You think say a joking?"
Ken tried to intervene.

"Where Earva gone, me say? You don't know?"
The young woman was still hesitant.

"Me want to find her, today, today ya."
The young woman appeared to be more prepared to give a response. But appeared to be only a fraction less uneasy at the questions being aimed at her by Ken.

"Mini and Maama move gone to 23 Charles Street. It is just 'round there so."
She gave a gesture of the right hand to indicate the general direction to the house.

"Me can show you where it is."
Lize didn't wait. She had already started her waddling away from the house. She had not waited to learn the name and number of the street. She was clear about the direction and seemed to gain speed in her steps and continued towards the street indicated by the young woman. Ken quickened his own steps in order to catch up with his mother. He had waited to receive the room number from the young woman. He anticipated a question from Lize as to the number of the rented room. Before she asked, he provided the information.

"Is number 40 she live at."
That detail was not critical for the moment because the news that Earva's mother from England was trying to find her had already been spread across the short distance between the two streets. There was not enough time to consider the clothes she was wearing or the state of her hair as Earva started out of the door of the room when her mother appeared in front of her. In a short moment, the physical space between them was usurped. They locked eyes. Their tears were spontaneous. Each entered the embrace of the other without a single word being spoken.

The protruding stomach of advanced pregnancy did not get into the way of their long embrace. The cry of both mother and daughter was audible from the neighbouring yard. There appeared to be a large congregation of uninvited spectators in the neighbouring gardens and veranda in the nearby streets. Inquisitive onlookers in rooms of the tenement house came to stand nearby in an attempt to watch the unfolding scene. They watched the close embrace. Earva was known to be a resident in the yard but the pregnant woman was a stranger to their eyes. Ken surveyed the faces and his gaze fell upon Maama. She was standing outside in the yard amongst the other tenants of the house. She was a young woman of slender physical build and dark complexion. They were cousins on the Moodie side of the family from Montpelier. Maama's parents were from Barnes Yard and they had grown up together in the district. They had been schoolmates and her sisters and brothers were of similar age to Bibs and Ken and the other Riggan children.

Earva had packed all her belongings into a large leather grip and three or four large plastic bags. Ken carried the large brown leather grip to the booth of the car. He placed the case in the car and quickly returned to collect the remaining luggage. Lize had reluctantly released her daughter from the embrace and returned to sit in the back seat of the car. For the first time since she had arrived in the city she became aware of being physically tired. She noticed the warm heat of the early afternoon sun. She kept her eyes focused on her teenage daughter across the yard. It was nearly four years since she had last seen her in the flesh.

Earva went to speak to her roommate. She handed over her keys and then said her good bye to other people she had come to know in the time of residing in the room shared with Maama. The interest in the pregnant woman and the shapely brown skinned teenage girl had largely passed and there was now only the gaze of the residents who also lived in the yard. The doors of the car slammed shut and the engine and sound of manual gears blended into a rhythm of the road that continued for the duration of the return journey westward from Montego Bay to Montpelier in Hanover. For the moment at least Lize's mind could rest at ease. Seven of her eight children were again safely under her wings. She would not worry about Bibs who had remained with her husband in England. There was only one remaining worry in her mind now and that was to know the exact date when her ninth child would make its appearance. The unborn child was putting more pressure on her bladder. She asked the car driver to pull in at the next public building they passed for her to relieve herself.

Chapter Six

Flying the Nest

The long distance correspondence by airmail between Ron in Britain and his wife on the island continued after her return. Some of the letters she wrote captured the extremities of her feelings for him. There were those times when she tried desperately to appeal to his sense of a united family living together again under one roof. This was the strongest of values she held about her family. When she reflected upon their many years together Lize felt a deep yearning in the soul for her husband. She wanted him to be present once again, in her life and in the guidance and support for their children. When letter after letter failed to bring about the end she had in mind for him the help of the children was solicited. Each child was encouraged by Lize to put pen to paper with words to persuade their father to return home to them on the island. The more Ron put up resistance to the request, the more the words rolled off his wife's pen and each have a very clear intent.

Ron continued to live the life of a single man in Britain. He had moved into a rented single room only a few months following the return home of Lize and baby Jimmy. He had made a promise to his wife to continue to work for a few more years in order to save some money. He would then return home to the island. He continued to meet his obligation to provide financial support to his wife and dependant children. But the visits to the public houses in the company of friends and workmates had returned in earnest following the departure of Lize. The taste for pleasures also returned as a feature of his life. It was only after the persistence of the letters from his wife and children and, the insistence by his sister Lillian in Walsall that Ron agreed to return home. A letter to confirm the date of his passage was sent ahead while his sister took up every opportunity to visit Walsall Market to buy items of clothing, shoes, kitchen and dining wares. The large freight was also packed with the items of furniture, the dismantled bed and wardrobe that were owned by Ron. As the date of his departure arrived, Ron worked his period of notice at the factory and said goodbye to family and friends in Walsall.

The arrival of Ron at the family home was long anticipated and the journey to Kingston Harbour was headed by Vandley and Denzil with a strong party of their male friends. They had no trouble in hiring a local truck before heading off to the capital city at dusk on the date given from their father's letter. He had arrived and waited in the arrival bay of the Harbour with returnees coming back to the island from Britain and America in particular. The boys locate their father among the bodies of men, women and children. Vandley was almost too anxious to see his father after waiting nearly ten years for this moment to arrive. He was only seven years old when Ron left the island for Britain in September 1957. The anticipation was too much for him as he forged his way forward through the crowd without even stopping to think about the others who had travelled with him. He had seen a passport sized photo of Ron and was confident he would be able to spot him in the crowd even from a distance. Some of the faces under his persistent stare were almost familiar to him, at least for a moment. But as he looked closer they appeared to become less so. Perhaps his father hadn't arrived as promised and he thought about sharing his new doubt with the others who he expected to be close behind him. When he looked around there was not a single face behind or beside him whom he recognised. He wondered where his brother and their party of friends were for a brief moment but went no further with that thought.

"Vandley, where you gone?"

He recognised Denzil's voice.

"You see him yet?"

Denzil's response was almost complete when Vandley wheeled away.

"Yes man, him come. See him over there so".

Vandley was heading towards his father.

"Is you is me father? A so you did look?"

"And what you name?"

"Me a you son."

Vandley continued with a laugh.

"Me name Roxy. You no 'memba me?"

Ron's gaze was on his over excited son. He smiled broadly and was obviously pleased to be reintroduced to his son.

"Is oofa pickney you?" Ron directed the question at Denzil as he stood next to his brother.

The laughter of the friends gave a hint of the identity to Ron.

"And you a Denny?"

"Yes sir, and me a you son too."

Ron embraced his sons for a moment. He felt pleased that they had now grown into young men. Each stood taller than their father with the first spout of facial hair already present. It was Vandley who secured the small handheld case from his father's grasp and offered to navigate him through the waiting crowd to the waiting truck. They would begin the journey home once more through the early hours from Kingston before they would reach Hanover.

The chattering and questioning continued during the journey home to the district. Most of the boys sat in the back of the truck amongst the luggage under the tarpaulin cover. Ron sat in the front seat with the driver. Vandley had contested for a seat next to his father but lost that battle to his older cousin Twidley. He positioned himself in the back of the truck close to the glass screen at the back with his eyes focussed on the side of his father's head under the felt hat. Occasionally, he met and returned Ron's gaze as he turned his head to peer into the darkness behind the passenger screen.

"Is so the man did short?"

The mocking response of his friend Comfy was lost on Vandley.

"You never know say a so him did short?", interrupted Dee.

"No, me never remember him like that. Me used to think say him was taller and big with nuff hair 'pon him head and 'pon him face."

"No sir, that man always short".

Comfy was starting to believe that he was the only one who remembered Ron by his appearance before he left the island nearly ten years ago.

"How you 'memba him, Comfy, if you is the same age as me?"

Vandley's enquiry brought others into the questioning of Comfy's memory.

"Is lie him a tell bout him "memba Ron", Dee was clearly siding with Vandley.

"I was a big man when him go'wa, around eleven year old.

The friends laughed at comfy.

He continued in his defence.

"When that man left and go a foreign I did know. Me na tel no lie. Me "memba him good, good.""

The conversation went on but without any of the other boys really believing that Comfy could really retain such a clear memory of Ron's appearance from a decade ago. The party arrived home after around four hours and had unloaded Ron's luggage from the truck to the house in next to no time. While most of the party disappeared into the break of day, Ron's wife and children and grandchildren greeted him as he made his entry into the house. Lize's heart felt glad as her husband slept during mid morning. She felt at ease with herself. The unity of her family had been restored for the first time in a decade and she hoped in her heart that Ron would feel the same contentment as she had.

During the next week Ron became reacquainted with the young men and women who had grown up in the time while he was away. Ken visited frequently but was unable to remain for any more than a few days at a time. He then had to bid his father and mother goodbye and set off to the parish of the church where he was serving as the assistant pastor to an older Minister. Ron commented on how Jimmy and Floyd and grand daughter Melva had grown quickly in the two and a half years since he had last seen them. He met his youngest son for the first time and couldn't agree on who it was in the family that the boy took his resemblance from.

The atmosphere of the full family home was happy although cramped with the sheer number of bodies who were present constantly, especially during the daytime. There were groups of friends visiting whom he had come to associate with each of Ken, Earva, Vandley and Denzil. The readjustment to family life was not proving easy for Ron and he struggled to assume any real authority over the household. Lize already assumed that role and whether by design or choice, this would be the destination for many years yet. The philosophy on conduct and discipline under Lize's roof was crystal clear and it was often repeated on each occasion that she felt it was necessary to administer corporal punishment for any behaviour of which she disapproved.

"If any of you want to live in my house, you follow my rules." Lize reaffirmed.

"Nobody should take things that don't belong to them. And don't start fight with other people's pickney." she warned.

"I don't like liars. Me don't want any of my pickney them to tell lies and cuss bad words under my roof." So oonu better understand. And who can't hear must feel."

She reaffirmed, "None a oonu don't bring girlfriend or boyfriend inna this house."

"As long as all a oonu have manners we will all live together under this roof."

The rules of Lize's house applied to her children, grandchildren and for that matter, it applied to everyone who cared to enter under the roof of her house. They applied to the young as well as to the old. On the matter of manners and respect she did not make any exception. When the rules were violated, the specially cut leather belt would make its appearance without fail. There was not even a faint chance that Lize could ever be accused of sparing the rod and spoiling any of her children. Ron had been back at home for a few months and had decided he wanted to raise and sell life stock of pigs, goats and cows. This he would combine with some small-scale farming on the piece of land they had purchased from the money earned in Britain. He had noticed that the primary industries of commercial plantation farming, road cutting and maintenance work had almost disappeared. The generation of his age group had become largely redundant by the absence of those early labour intensive industries.

The politics of the island had also undergone major changes with the coming of political independence from Britain's colonial governance. The end of the busy decade of the 1960s was approaching. His children were growing up fast and Ron was quite uncertain as to where he would fit into the landscape. He had worked in Britain for nearly a decade and had become accustomed to the ebb and flow of metal foundry and copper refinery. There was a certain discipline to work in British factories with 6am start until 4pm for shift work. Over time he had become accustomed to that environment and its routines.

He was approaching the age of forty-five. There was a definite unwillingness by his body to respond to the demand being made to cut and till the ground. He had purchased a few life stocks. But as the older children begun to move on to find apprenticeship training and work Ron began to harbour some serious doubt about whether he could return to the lifestyle of substance farming that he had left behind a decade earlier.

He conversed with his wife.

"Lize, you notice how things change up here now?" He enquired.

She provided him with a response.

"When me did come back me notice how the place start to get built up. You don't see some of the house them that people building all over the area?"

Ron had noticed.

"Me see the new basic school building out a ball ground. Them really start to build up the place now?" he asked.

"And you don't notice say them widen the road and asphalt it from Sandy Bay to Montpelier as well?" Lize continued in response to her husband's questioning.

"But them need to chop down some a them trees that hanging over the road down by Little Level, near Miss Carrow." Ron continued with the conversation as he lay across the foot of the bed.

Ron continued, "But people not farming like them used to do before? Me did think say people still plant food and carry them to sell at market. Me surprise to see all these little shops open and selling things like pack rice, and flour and other things like that."

Lize had listened patiently to her husband. She had detected his anxiety. She hoped that her responses expressed the new reality of the many visible areas of change on the island.

"Yes, little Jamaica is not like the way how you did leave it. Everything a change up and them even have black people a take part in voting and politics now."

Lize noted that the island was no longer a British colony. It could elect its own political leaders and had abandoned the use of the Imperial currency of pound, shilling and pence. Following its independence from Britain the island adopted the Jamaican dollar as the national trading currency. A new era of two party politics had emerged onto the landscape of the island and they were now attracting loyal and partisan following. Many issues that both Lize and Ron felt to be of importance on the island in general and in the districts of Montpelier and Cascade in particular entered into the conversation.

Ron continued, "Lize, I don't think I can work the land again, you know? The place a get too hot and me can't afford to pay people to work anymore."

Lize responded sharply.

"But you only just come back, man, and you have to get used to the country again."

Ron reasserts, "All of them boys said the country is getting harder for poor people to get work and mind them family. No work is here for anybody. And especially when you can't read and write good."

Ron's tone of resignation raised a strong concern in Lize. She would not try to force the issue just now. She attempted to consolidate on the concerns of her husband.

"Yes, the country change, but people still find ways to live and mind them family. And that is all that we want, eh?"

She was hoping to receive Ron's consent.

"We don't need much, except we food and clothes. We have a nice piece of land here with everything on it. We have bananas, breadfruit, coconut, cane, ackee, and we can plant anything else that we want. We don't own anybody rent and we don't owe anybody any debt. So what else we could want here?"

Ron agreed, at least in part, but felt the need to repeat his concern that the country was getting harder for the poorer people.

During the following weeks Ron returned to the same concerns and when he showed no real interest in taking on board the advice of his wife it soon became a question of just when he would decide to head off to Britain again? Lize made it clear that she no longer wished to return to Britain at any time in the future. The older of the children would soon be able to make their own way in this world and while the younger ones were still growing up, she had no intention of leaving them again. Her patience was ebbing away with each new hint of a desire by Ron to leave his family behind once more and return to Britain.

He was not surprised by the next utterance from his wife.

"Listen man, if you think the dirty work and cold inna Britain a call you, then you go back to it."

The resigned look on her face made her feelings clear to Ron.

"I staying right here in me house with me pickney them." Ron knew his wife better than anyone else and so far as the matter was concerned he alone would make the final decision. That time soon arrived and it was not long before the arrangement for Ron's departure was made. Ken was instructed by his father to book the passage from the new Norman Manley International Airport in Kingston to London. The journey time to Britain would be completed in a day. He said his good byes to his wife before leaving home. She did not travel to the airport with the small party of the four oldest children and she did not bother to watch as her husband disappeared on his walk from her view before boarding the hired car for the airport.

The relationship between Lize and her older children would begin to change as they again adjust to life without Ron. Ken visited his mother from his church base in the east of the island. Bibs sent money for maintaining her two children regularly at the end of each month. Vandley was now serving as an apprentice joiner and carpenter with a well-established building contractor. Earva was at home but without a job and she would soon decide that it was now her turn to fly the family nest.

"Mim, me want to ask you something. You hear?"

Lize gazed towards her daughter's face.

"One a me friends said we can find work in Kingston with a woman, if we go up there."

The response by her mother was immediate.

"And you want to go up there for it?"

Earva took a slight evasive step backwards. She was already feeling fearful that Lize would not agree that she should be going.

"How you know say the work is there for you? You ever go to Kingston yet?"

The disapproval by her mother was undisguised.

"Look how far where Kingston is?"

Earva tried to intervene, "But Mim, no work is not in Montpelier for me to get, and other people go to Kingston and find work already."

Lize recognised that look of equal determination on her daughter's face. She had been able to observe her at close quarters during the past three years and could be confident in her growing maturity. She also knew that in another year or so Earva would be entering her twenties.

"You will need to think about this very carefully because as far as I know, Kingston is not a nice place. People will kill you and when them done them will throw your body a door for dogs to eat."

"Mim, me think about it already and me want to go."

The door was slammed shut behind the young woman as she turned away from her mother's bedroom. Lize recognised that her children were growing up fast and she had become resigned to watching them go on their way, whether she gave her approval or not. Ken was also present in the room and had overheard the conversation but did not intervene. His head remained still on his folded forearms in a slumber across the width of the bed. After Earva had left he changed position and advice his mother to let his sister go if she wanted to. He reminded Lize that Earva was now a grown woman and it was not for her to tell her what to do anymore. In the morning Lize would again restart the conversation with her daughter about her intention of going to Kingston. On this occasion, she was more concerned to alert the young woman to some potential dangers that may lay ahead. She did not make any further attempt to instruct her on what to do. Lize gave her daughter the full blessing and added some money to assist with travel and living until she found a job in the capital city.

Chapter Seven

Rebel

The enforced return from England by Lize may have been caused by a worry over the six children she had left behind on the island nearly four years earlier. The youngest of these children was Barry and in the twelve months that Lize had returned she had noticed that a trait of stubbornness was present in the boy's character. She wondered whether her absence during some of his formative years had left any long-term emotional bearing on her fourth son. The boy had not directed much of his attention towards her. In her mind she had noted the sharp contrast with the friendly attention given to her by Noreen who was nearly twelve and two years older than her younger brother. Denzil was two years older than Noreen and he showed himself to be very happy in the company of his mother. The two older children who were still at home, Earva and Vandley, had also built up close relationships with Lize. Their grandmother Estry and cousin Twidley occupied a small neighbouring wooden house that was built slightly adjacent to the larger house.

Barry seemed to spend most of his time in the small house with his grandmother. He also showed less interest in attending church with his mother and the others while the verbal reports Lize received from school gave further cause for concern. She continued to make the effort to develop a relationship with Barry while giving care and attention to her two youngest sons, besides the grandchildren she had brought back from England, Melva and Floyd.

Barry was born only a year before Ron left for Britain in the autumn of 1957. He had not got to know his father properly. Ron had returned to the island in 1966 but stayed for only a short period of only six months before returning to Britain alone. Barry was around ten years old at the time. When Lize left for Britain in 1961, he was still very young. It was perhaps true that he experienced the worse effects from the disruption in his relationship with both Lize and Ron during his formative years. As the youngest of the children left on the island, he would have picked up the uncertainty from the others about whether or not they should follow eldest sister Bibs to join Ron in Britain. He would probably not have been consulted on any first or final decision made on the matter. So when Lize returned to the island in mid 1960s, Barry would have already begun to feel emotionally detached from her. When she returned with the younger children and grandchildren, her full attention would have been taken up with matters beside Barry's emotional development.

At aged eleven, Barry had already begun to display a strong aptitude for stubbornness. He was not the model child that his mother had hoped for and neither was he seen as having ambitions in the mould of Ken or Vandley. His older brothers were already graduating into mature young men of twenty-one and seventeen years of age respectively. Ken was about to be married and settled into life as a minister within the church. Vandley was undertaking his apprenticeship training and would soon be on his way to a life in the island capital of Kingston. Earva would soon be gone with Denzil set to follow in due course. All around him there had always been changes and upheavals. The others now being of age, Barry inherited the mantle of the oldest son present in the yard. But this would also mean more exposure under the eyes and authority of Lize. She had established her method of bringing up children and while those ahead of him endured the discipline of their mother, this would not go unchallenged by this most tempestuous child. When the orders came down from Lize, more often than not, they were not followed willingly by Barry. When the rules of the house were laid down, more often than not, they were broken. Chalk and cheese had nothing on this duo.

Against the backdrop of the turbulence of the island's urban political violence and the surge in reggae music and ganja smoking as a focus for young people, Barry chose to demonstrate his manhood by rebelling against all the things that his mother stood for. He refused to attend Sunday school from the age of twelve or thirteen. He showed no real interest in education except for the open or coded message in the records of reggae artists. Barry became part of the crowd of friends that Lize spent all her life detesting and avoiding. At aged fourteen and before the end of his compulsory schooling, he achieved an unwelcome family first by being permanently expelled from school for retaliating physically against a teacher who was about to administer corporal punishment for some misdemeanour. The report from the headteacher at the school would represent the final straw for Lize and she wasted not time in letting her son know exactly what she thought of him.

"You have no manners; you have no respect and I will pray to God for you."

Barry retorted, "All the while is only me one who you want to hold quarrel with. Why is always me? Is only me who don't have manners and respect?"

The full ferocity of her tongue was bent on her son.

"I want you out of this yard. Go 'way, you John Crow. You have no manners."

Barry kept at a safe distance away from his mother as they continue to exchange angry words.

"You think I want to live inna your house? I will go a street and let other people put I up."

"So go on, you dirty John Crow. You old ram goat. Me tears will react against you. Bad blessing will follow you. Go from me yard." As Lize advanced in the direction of her son, and all the time searching the ground for a stick with which to launch her assault, Barry retreated hurriedly from the yard.

It was not the first time that they had a very public quarrel. Lize had attempted to establish dominance over the challenges presented by her son for some time. She tried the well-used methods of the whip from earlier years. The hard talk made no real avail on the behaviour of Barry. She attempted to hold up her older sons as good models of obedient and respectful children but to no apparent avail. She asked older male members of the family to speak to Barry on her behalf in a further attempt to bring him under her discipline but again with no return for the effort. And when everything else appeared to have failed then it was the turn of corporal punishment. The physical size and strength of her son always presented a special challenge to her average sized and largely under weight body. But Lize has never been put off by the prospect of a personal challenge. In time she would apprehend him with the help of older boys in the yard.

"Whiz", went the vibrating sound of the stiff leather belt as it collided with Barry's back.

His shout under the sting of the belt had become well rehearsed.

" Lord, Mim, that is like a gun pincher."

He struggles to free himself from the tightened grip of her hand.

Barry's punishment was meted out under the full glare of his older brothers and watching friends.

Wizz! went another stroke of the belt.

"And that one is like a spanner." He struggles but can't free himself.

"Lord, Mim, let me go. Let me go now. Let me go."

Barry's running commentary on each lash he received from the belt wielded by Lize continued on each occasion until the years of his early teens.

Barry was growing up in the district with a crowd of local teenagers who were becoming very conscious of the adverse social and economic position occupied by teenagers on the island. They adopted the dreadlock hairstyle of uncut and uncombed plaited hair. They adopted the styles of clothes in the colours of red, green and gold. They cultivated and smoke marijuana. They collected the emblems of the Rasta man. Barry understood and repeated the challenging words of defiance coming over the airwaves by reggae artists and bands led by Jacob Miller, Burning Spears, Bob Marley and the Wailers. The direct literal and metaphorical words of the most popular songs were well rehearsed by youth across the island as the indigenous recording industry expanded from the urban ghettoes of Kingston. The influence of youth was rising in a challenge to the status quo of older people, church and the law.

Barry made it abundantly clear to his mother that he and his friends would not spend their Saturday evenings in preparation for the regular Sunday service. They were of a new generation who were quite willing to challenge the system of the island's social and cultural order. Instead of serving God they would threaten to burn down churches. They did not respect the traditional leaders of church, school, politicians or wealth. The shout of their defiance was for "Jah to Guide and Protect I". They found a popular outlet in the ganja smoke filled weekend dance hall. Lize soon worked out that this would never be a winning battle. Her son was much more inclined to respond to the advice of Bob Marley than he was to show obedience to his mother. She did not accept but understood that the island and its challenging new generations were changing.

Chapter Eight

New Beginnings

It was Ron's intention to return to England for a further period of five years. He had made it clear to his wife that he was returning to Britain to work in order to secure the financial future of the family. Before he left the island he asked his brothers Moodie and Dawz to keep an eye on the small stock of a few herds of cow, goats, pigs and chickens. The financial proceeds generated from these animals and by the fruits of his land should go towards the support of Lize and the dependant children he had left behind. The small family stock was fully stretched to support his family through the cost of schooling and maintenance and a certain frostiness soon returned between Lize and her husband. As a consequence, the financial support from Ron quickly dried up and it was left largely to the older children to contribute to the upkeep of the family. After a further four years passed Ron had yet again turned back on his words of promise to return to his wife on the island.

By the reports received by Lize, her husband had returned to his previous life of working hard and then spending his earning in public houses and being footloose with women. The uncompromising pen wielded by Lize made clear that the durable ties of their marriage and children were being put under strain once too often. The solution she believed was simple: *'either the duck left the pond or, the pond should leave the duck.'* She put her solution to him and asked that he choose. The relationship between Lize and her older children would also begin to change as they adjusted to an uncertain future without Ron.

Ken completed his period of theological training during the year after his father's departure from the island and he was assigned the full pastoral leadership of a church in the parish of St Mary, to the east of the island. He had also got engaged to a young woman, Eunice Wright, who was one of the students on the training programme at the college. Their wedding followed shortly afterwards in the absence of Ron but with the full blessing of Lize. Ken visited his mother from his church base frequently, and providing her with both financial and emotional support. Bibs would also send money to her mother to meet the cost of maintaining the two oldest grandchildren, Melva and Floyd. Vandley excelled as a keen young apprentice joiner and carpenter with a well-established building contractor and he too was able to contribute some financial support to the family coffers. Younger brother Denzil took on the duty of subsistence farming hand under the guidance of uncles Moodie and Dawz. They each contributed to the maintenance of the family.

Around the time of his eighteenth birthday, it was Vandley's turn to inform Lize of his intention to join Earva in the capital city. The unintended consequence was to trigger a further pattern of chain migration as younger brothers Denzil and Barry also followed the same path to Kingston from Hanover during the next three years. The trend breaker was younger sister Noreen who settled instead for the convention of church and marriage in the district while remaining close by her mother.

Eldest sister Bibs fulfilled her pledge and returned to the island from Britain in 1970. The two older grandchildren, Melva and Floyd, were joined by younger sister Debbie on the return of their mother who went to settle with her husband in the central parish of Clarendon. There was further addition to the nest of the family during the decade as the number of grandchildren multiplied quickly by the contribution of a third daughter, Erica, by Bibs. Ken contributed sons Henry, Junior and Rohan before daughter Kareen arrived. Vandley added three daughters with a young woman in Kingston, Paula, Donna and Karen. Denzil weighed in with a set of twins, Tanya and Troy with Rudell Blackwood in Kingston, before consolidating his love interest with Geta Allison and producing sons Torry, Tyrone and Kevin. Noreen continued to live in the district and with her husband, William Mc Nish, and they added sons Dale, Sean and Nordley before the arrival of daughter Nicolette. Barry had also begun to make his contribution to the family with the arrival of his first son, Chandale at the turn of the new decade of the 1980s. The clutch of offsprings provided Lize with a glimpse of future generations from the seeds of Riggan, Moodie, Patterson and Bartley families.

In a period of quite serious social, political and economic instability on the island, a further trend towards migration overseas became part of the ambition of many Jamaican families. The mass unemployment caused by the decline in traditional rural labour driven industries of forestry and commercial plantation farming had the effect of speeding up the movement of new generations to urban ghettos. The skills possessed by Vandley in carpentry and joinery came in very useful when he started working at MacGibbon Furniture Company on the Walton Park Road in Kingston. They made household furniture such as dining tables, bed frames, wardrobes, settees, chairs and bathroom cabinets.

The low pay from his hard work did not please Vandley and he soon became convinced that he could do the same and perhaps even better for himself. He had developed a spirit for enterprise and that was soon translated into his taking on side orders and filling them by setting up a makeshift workshop in the garden of the tenement house he shared with Earva and Denzil. As the volume of orders coming to him increased from friends and family Vandley was persuaded to quit the day job and make a proper fist of his own small furniture making business in the capital city. For a few years at least things seemed to have gone well with an increasing number of large orders secured from some established furniture retailers and smaller shops. The family shared the benefits from Vandley's labour. On the occasions when things did go wrong in the lives of her children, Lize provided a continuous support by way of her letters and advice. They were encouraged to follow the ethos of a sharing and caring family and so they stayed together and looked out for each other.

Near the close of the decade of the 1970s a further phase of chain migration was set in motion within the family. It had come near the end of the year 1978 when there was a decisive intervention made by Lillian on behalf of her brother, Ron. She had continued to maintain active communication with Lize by letter while keeping a close eye on her brother. It was Lillian who would ensure that some of the loose change that fell from Ron's fortnightly pay pocket found its way to Lize on the island. The mandatory retirement age for British industrial workers was on the near horizon for Ron and Lize had already given consideration to whether she should again make all the running to reconcile with her husband. She had long ruled out divorce on grounds that this would not bode well for her children or grandchildren. As a committed Pentecostal Christian who was still living in the nest of her husband's family in the district of Montpelier, the road to the family court did not hold much appeal for her. It was now almost twelve years since Ron had walked out the door to return to Britain.

Lize shared the information received from Lillian with her eldest son.

"Ken, your father want me to go back to Britain before him retire. Him ask him sister to write me a letter last week and ask me if I would consider coming back with the two last boys."

For many years her eldest son had stood closely by her side in the absence of his father, and Lize wanted to receive any view that he might hold on the issue. Ken was surprised by the content of the information received from his father.

"So him not looking to come back home? Him wants to die in England? Ron is turning old man now and him should be looking to come home out of the cold"

Ken did not feel inclined to hold any sympathy for his father's sentiments to have his wife return to Britain.

Lize replied, "I already ask him whether him intend to come back home, and him say him want to come home, but after him retire."

Lize hoped that her son would make his own position clear.

She continued, "And it look like say him still have women eating him out, so if me don't go back then them will only send back him bones inna box to we."

Ken recognised the anxiety held by his mother.

"How much more times he expect you to fix problems for him? Him have to agree to come home first, and then you should go over there and bring him back so that he can receive his pension and enjoy the final years of his life. "

After a pause, Ken probed his mother further.

"Is Ron prepared to do that?"

Lize responded almost instantly.

"Me been considering the situation and, to tell you the truth, I not sure what to do. I want to talk it over with the others too."

A short pause followed as Ken focused his gaze on his mother's face. She was now past fifty years old and he became sharply conscious of the signs of her loneliness and vulnerability for the first time.

"Bibs think I should go back to him. And Earva, and Vandley them think say I should go to."

Ken again looked directly in the face of his mother, but without seeking any haste in her response.

"What about Denzil and Noreen? What they say?"

She continued, "well Denzil him say him will agree with whatever me and the others say. But as you know, me have Denzil's two twins here with me so if me leave that is bound to affect them too."

Ken sought to reassure his mother that even without his speaking to Denzil, he was certain he would not ask her to remain on the island just for the sake of maintaining his children.

"I'm sure that the twins, Tanya and Troy, will be all right. Them can go to live with their mother or even stay with Noreen or Bibs."

A family consensus was established between Lize and her children. The process of applying for new passports to travel to Britain would take a bit longer than was anticipated. Neither of the two youngest children had previously possessed a passport and in the case of Jimmy, he was born in England and a copy of the birth certificate had to be applied for from London. Lize completed the requisite form with the surname spelling 'Riggan'. There was a long delay before a letter was received without the birth certificate. It contended that the record of the registry office for new births in Walsall could not find any child by the surname

71

stated on the form. In fact they had found a birth registered for the date and hospital but the surnames were inconsistent. It was recorded as 'Riggon'. There were several letters by Lize to plead that the inconsistency in the different letters of the 'a' and the 'o' was merely as a result of a recording error. The civil servants administering the matter in Walsall did not agree with her and after a while she was given the ultimatum of either making a challenge in the courts in London to change the recording of Jimmy's surname or, accept the disputed birth certificate. She was advised that the name could be legally amended by deed poll. There would be a cost to her from the exercise of either option. Lize was a practical woman and she opted to return to Britain on a passport bearing the surname of 'Mrs Riggan', while her sons were recorded as 'Riggon'. She hoped that some time in the future the surname of all her children would be written in the same way. They returned to the English Midlands in time for the new decade of the 1980s.

Earva had left the island for Grand Cayman in 1976. She got married to a young Guyanese man and remained in Cayman for a few years. She later moved to America. In April 1980 Ken also departed the island for the western Canadian Province of Alberta. Within a further period of six years, the chain of family migration also took Vandley and Denzil to North America. Barry had also added daughter Juliene and son Richie to the family before he also departed the island. The oldest grand children, Melva, Floyd and Debbie went back to England, while almost all the other grand children were headed for a new life in Canada or the United States before the end of the decade. The exception from these events was again Noreen and her children who remained on the island.

Chapter Nine

Push and Pull

In the case of Vandley the critical push from the island came when the business that he had established fell upon difficult times. He may well have been guilty of some rather poor judgement in his choice of business partners. As a man of exceptionally kind disposition towards granting aid to family and friends he appeared to push himself to the limit to grant favours. As a consequence the bad credits mounted up and were equalled only by the high number of new entry onto the payroll. The workshop had inadvertently become a dive to many young hangers on who contributed nothing of any real worth to the viability of the business. Soon the creditors came calling and when there was no sign of a sustainable cash flow they sent the bailiffs in to value the capital assets of machinery and stock. The advice of his mother was never far away.

> *My dear son,*
> *I received your letter and was very concerned to hear you say that your business was not performing well. Son, you must be careful not to let friends and strangers take what you have and*

then go bring you down. Remember say Kingston people them don't stay like Montpelier people. Them will take away what you have and then turn around and put them gun on you. I know you mean well when you say you want to carry on with the business so as to not layoff your workers. But listen to me, son, you can't put their interest in front of your own. You is a stranger to them. You must be careful about who you get into business with. You must mind. You hear what me tell you say? You must mind what you doing.

Take care until I hear from you again.
Your Loving Mother,
Lize

The end of that operation came about quite quickly after that and without the presence of Lize nearby to provide counsel Vandley was left alone all at sea without a paddle. He then took a bold step of venturing to Canada where he joined elder brother Ken in the western province of Alberta. Vandley overcame the grip of the uncompromising Canadian winter to settle into a life of temporary work. When the period of his landing was expired, he felt the need to take a chance and violate the terms of his immigrant status by going to ground in order to continue work in the country. He survived the sweeps of immigration authority long enough to re-establish contact on the island with the young woman and the three girls. The period away had a quite adverse effect on the relationship with the young woman, who had by now found a new lover. After a further period of around three years in Canada, Vandley was still keen to reconcile the situation of his family and the young woman was invited to join him in Alberta.

In hindsight this did not turn out to be a good move. The attempted reconciliation ended in failure with the young woman returning to the island alone. Shortly after this Vandley was conspicuously caught out in a dawn raid on his rented house by Canadian Immigration officials. He was apprehended and made subject to deportation back to the island. For the first time in his life, Vandley would be alone without the support of a close family network. He absorbed the extreme pressures of Kingston for nearly two years, without the young woman and his three girls, before he was presented with a further opportunity to steal away off the island again. This time his destination would be the Big Apple.

Many difficult situations are sometimes overcome, not by any grand strategy but by a stroke of good luck. That was the case with Vandley after he had gaffed his way through the airport custom control at Kennedy's Airport in New York. He had only just arrived from the island. It was late in the evening and he needed a taxi to go to Earva's house at an address in Brooklyn. After failing to wave down two or three cabs that had sped by, a woman driver pulled up near the arrival lounge.
"Jump in sugar, and tell me just where you headin'. Is it Queens or Brooklyn for you tonight?"
She was a bright spark and after a long stop over at Miami for the connecting flight to New York, Vandley could use the friendly voice of this New Yorker.
"Where you luggage, sugar. You' a lithe traveller. I can see that."
He had already got into the passenger side of the cab when she slammed the empty car boot shut and climbed in and gave the pedal under her right foot a firm press.

"So where you say we heading, darlin'? Tell me so I can get into the right lane here."

Vandley responded, "Brooklyn, Vandalia Avenue."

"And where in the hell is that, sugar? Do you know, cause I sure don't!"

As far as Vandley was concerned, the driver was from New York. She should know where the place was.

"You don't know where it is, lady?"

The driver smiled at him.

"Hell no, ain't never been called a Lady before. You island boys sure do have good manners now, don't you? You can call me Mary, now. That's my name, sugar. And what's yours?

A further swivel of the steering wheel at the intersection and they were heading into the lane with the 'Brooklyn Bridge' sign overhead. Mary was running on adrenalin and when she slowed to indicate right at the intersection, Vandley could see the name of the avenue given from his sister's address.

"Is there so it is." He indicated by pointing his right hand.

Mary was already part way through her question of asking which 'apartment block'.

"Sixteen. Is apartment number sixteen."

"Well sugar, let me see the paper you got there." Mary had no trouble deciphering the number 16.

"Oh yes, you're right. Number sixteen it is."

She surveyed the vicinity of the yard near the entry to the apartment.

"Got anyone inside to meet you, sugar?"

"Yes. My sister is there. She should be home now."

It was after ten thirty in the evening but the Brooklyn sky was still high. The clothes he had selected eight hours earlier were staring to feel sweaty. Vandley wanted to go inside.

Mary went to the intercom. She pressed the small red button.

"Buzz Buzz."

"No response, sugar. Try it again."

Three or four further push against the buzzer brought no response. The thought that the address might be wrong went through his head at least a few times.

"Like no body home, now. You got anywhere else to stop?"

"No. This is the right address. My sister live here. Maybe she is sleeping."

"Buzz. Earva. Buzz. Earva you home?"

She could see the slight anxiety on his face.

"Well it don't look good, now." Mary stepped backward from under the roof to survey the upper side of the apartment.

"Better you get a number and call her. You got her number?"

"I don't think so, you know." He felt for the missing item in the pocket on his shirt and then in the pockets of the trousers. It was late by now and Mary switched the cab light to: "Off Duty". She felt in a generous mood and she made him an offer and he did not refuse.

Vandley was in New York three full days before he made contact with his sister. They spoke by phone and when Mary came back home from her day's work, the cab light was again switched to 'Off Duty'. They travelled again to Earva's apartment. Mary met the mystery sister and was not at all shy to share a joke with her at Vandley's expense. He continued to stay with Mary and after a few weeks, he initiated a discussion with Mary about the taxi business. He was a little surprised when she suggested that they could share the driving and the cost of the vehicle. It was not her personal vehicle, but she had kept it on a driver lease agreement. She would show him the routes and teach him the business. In return, he would pay to her an agreed weekly amount and take on the early morning and late night run which she was not too crazy about.

During the next two years the driving partnership between them worked quite amicably. They shared an apartment and all the main costs for renting and food. They shared the driving and the repair of the vehicle. The main areas of disagreement between them came around the scheduling of the rota for early morning and weekend duty. Vandley insisted on alternating the rota. Mary would insist that since she was effectively his boss, then it was only fair that he should just go along with the programme. He was getting a bit fed up with what he felt was the unreasonableness of the whole thing and suggested that he could try to work up a similar arrangement between himself and a cab leasing firm without Mary. That didn't sound like a good plan to Mary and she let Vandley know. He didn't argue further but was resigned in his mind to sort out a separate deal for himself without her. When she found out about his plot, there was no holding back. He apologised for any misunderstanding. She didn't accept. The next time he went out in the cab and returned to the apartment, there were two suitcases left outside the doorway of the apartment with his name on them. The locks to the apartment door were changed and there was no response from the buzzer on the door. He was soon resigned to the faith. That was it. The relationship was now finished. He collected the items and went downstairs in the lift. The cases were placed in the booth of the cab and he returned to share the story with his friend who lived on the ground floor at the apartment. He returned to see Mary once or twice after he had secured his own apartment but things would never be the same again.

Some time after the split with Mary, he took up a *lease to drive* agreement of his own. In only a few months, the cab was badly damaged at the wing to the right near the passenger door following a road accident. The collision happened in broad daylight. Vandley was unhurt physically, but the woman passenger that he was transporting seemed quite badly shaken up. She was shaken and had asked for an ambulance. The young driver in the offending car was not visibly hurt but he seemed quite anxious to leave the scene before the police arrived. A small group of onlookers gathered near the damaged cars as they remained in their original position from the collision. The street was long and disappeared in the far distance. The cars were left positioned to the side of the carriageway. They could be passed quite easily and were not blocking the direct path of any other vehicle. Faces peeked out from behind curtains along the street. There were houses stretched along both sides of the street and interrupted by a liquor store and gas station on opposite sides of the road. In the milling of confusion caused by the collision, Vandley had not given much focus to the young driver involved. When he later glanced to the side in the direction of where the young driver had been standing, he realised that the driver had managed to disappear in the confusion. He had spoken to him only briefly to ask if he was all right and to have his driver detail and insurance papers ready before the ambulance arrived. The driver seemed concerned enough and had nodded in approval. He was black and spoke with a New York accent.

It was some time before the private registered ambulance arrived. The passenger was a fifty-seven year old African American female. She remained seated in the cab with the door closed and the window rolled down half way. They asked about the insurance details for the Cab Company and took other details from Vandley.

"And who is the driver for the other vehicle?" The eyes of the Paramedics surveyed the faces of the small attending crowd. They were largely black. There was no response on behalf of the young vehicle.

"I'm afraid we'll have to radio this one in. We'll need a photograph of the position of the two cars."

Vandley felt a little confused as to how the matter could be resolved when the other driver had already disappeared.

"What about the other driver?" Vandley felt obliged to ask, although he feared he already knew the answer to his own question.

"You'll have to move that car to the side of the next street." The paramedic was pointing at the yellow cab. He collected a form from his colleague after helping the female passenger into the wheelchair they had rolled from the back of the ambulance.

"Who gonna tell this to the police? Am I supposed to do all that?" Vandley was uncertain.

"Mr Riggan, you need to complete that form and take the part at the bottom with all your driving detail to the police. You should try to do so today, please." The blue light on top of the ambulance was set to flash but without the siren.

The paramedic continued, "And you should also get to a hospital and have yourself checked out. Looks like a mighty hard blow she took right there." The paramedic pointed to the head of the passenger as she was wheeled away from the scene of the collision.

The letter arrived from the insurance company. Vandley had been waiting for this. He was being asked to furnish more information about his agreement with the Taxi leasing company. The firm was the legal owners of the cab and Vandley had been told that they would handle any claim made against him by the passenger. It had been a few months now since the accident and he was beginning to feel that the tone of these letters was not at all supportive of his position. He was without a cab and therefore a livelihood. There was still no sign of the matter being brought to a close. It was now almost eight weeks since he was last able to earn a fare from the cab. He would go to see Earva again. Things were really getting him down. When it was over he would have to think hard about this whole driving business and the agreement with the company from where he leased the car. When matters were finally sorted, he felt it went against him. The insurance met the cost of the accident claim settled with the passenger, while the repair for the cab was passed on to Vandley. He was informed that the other vehicle involved in the accident was uninsured and the police were still unable to trace the driver of the stolen Mustang Convertible. There was nothing else that they could do on the matter. The next premium for the cab would also be increased as a result of the heavy claim just settled in favour of the passenger and the cost of the ambulance and, the hospital. This was a bad episode for Vandley and it was some considerable time before he would be back on his feet again.

Chapter Ten

Big Apple

When Vandley first arrived in New York there was a flutter of raw excitement running throughout his body and mind. He soon caught up with his good friend Lenny, who had arrived in the Big Apple some months earlier from Kingston. Vandley didn't like the unfamiliar taste of the bottle of Budweiser beer that his friend ordered. He fixed his full attention on Lenny and fired off a volley of burning questions.

"So what you been doing with yourself since you get up here, ole man? He asked his friend.

"Boy Vandley, things fast man, so you have to watch your steps and mind what you doing".

Lenny offered his friend a cigarette from an open box held in the pocket of his shirt before continuing.

"Is nuff man from back home who you find up here, man, but some a them just a hustle. Fast. And some just a cool for a while, man."

It was the way that Lenny punctuated the word 'Fast' that caught Vandley's attention.

"So is what them a do so fast, brother?

"Them a hustle, man."

"What them a hustle?"

Vandley wasn't sure whether he understood fully the intent with which his friend was speaking. He had in his mind an idea that this may have something to do with black market business but he decided not to pursue that particularly point further on this occasion. He had another subject in mind.

"So get the beer in no brother, is your round, ole man."

Lenny flicked out the pack of Benson 'n Hedges with just two remaining cigarettes showing.

Vandley made his order as the young female waitress moved passed their table.

"Two more of these beers, please."

She smiled and made a brief note on a small writing pad.

"Me hear say the work side slow in the trade. Things go so fe true?"

Lenny was quick with his reply.

"Boy from me come up ya me eyes don't see even one builders yard. Not even one, man."

"And so much damn buildings is here, man?" Vandley sip his beer more slowly this time around. He was hoping that his friend would have made some contacts in the building trade. They had worked at his workshop in Kingston for several years and he knew that his friend was as hard a worker as he was.

During the course of the conversation he was able to get some information about the different areas of the city where some other friends from the island were now residing. He noted down some telephone numbers on a piece of scrap paper left on the table. He was not too discouraged because of the reports his friend had provided on the building trade and in his mind he thought that he could do much better. He felt he had the skills and the experience for most of the work in the building and carpentry trade. If he was presented with the option of seeking work in the building trade and that of working in a high earning low labour intensity position, he would be quite prepared to take up the opportunity without a second thought. He well remembers the many hours spent speaking with Lenny about the fast routes he would take to make life in America. He had arrived only a few days and there was already doubt about how different the reality of life in New York City was appearing to be.

Five years in New York was all but a blurb. Everything had slipped by so quickly and the more he tried to re-run over his tracks the less clarity there was in his head. There was the job on a building site but that didn't last very long. The main foreman was also from the island originally. Vandley was hopeful of developing a close affinity when another friend from Kingston had first introduced him to Hubert Davis. But it just didn't happen. He felt the man was just too pushy and go on like he was 'American'. If you were two minutes late the threat to discipline was almost guaranteed.

"You was supposed to be on the site at eight o'clock. Try and remember that next time, ok?" Mr Davis would repeat.

He was definitely not charitable to his own islanders and in fact Vandley was starting to believe that the man didn't like people of his own colour! He thought about why the man behaving so awful with the Jamaicans on the site? And how comes he didn't seem to crack the whip in the same way for the Mexican and Latinos?

It didn't take long before the sword of the site foreman crossed Vandley.

"What happen brother, you can't see say is the wrong drill you using? You sure say you work in the building trade before?"

The comments were directed at a young Jamaican who looked un-nerved by Mr Davis. He shuffled around at the open tool bag in an attempt to make amends and to prevent the foreman from getting anymore crossed than he already was. Vandley stood in close proximity to the young man. The foreman returned to the error of the drill after a few seconds had passed.

"So pick up the bits them no man. Something is wrong with you today?"

Mr Davis continued to express his obvious annoyance.

He continued, "You can't find the right drill?"

His stare was still fixed on his prey.

"If something wrong with you then come off me site, man. Put down the tools them and leave, man. "

The young worker seemed hesitant to respond to the foreman.

Mr Davis persisted, "You don't hear what I say?"

One or two voices could be heard coming to the defence of the young man. He spoke faintly in his own defence.

"But Mr Davis, is just a simple mistake that you know sir. Just give I a chance no sir. Is beg I a beg you, you know, sir."

The plea didn't seem to be having the desired effect on Mr Davis.

"Is when them run street late a night and come straight onto the job in the morning without sleep that concern me more, you know."

Mr Davis was hoping to ensure that there was no more sympathy for the young man and against his action.

"Them full up themselves with all kind a street drugs and then come on the site fe cause accident."

After a short pause to allow another plea, Mr Davis issued another firm refusal and the young man began his walk towards the car park.

"But boss, him never do anything dangerous. So why you have to fire him like that?"

Vandley could sense the sharp resentment from the face of the site foreman.

"And is when you start here? He attempted to provide the answer to his own question. "Is last month, eh?"

He looked into Vandley's face without moving any part of his body other than his pivoting head while the stare remained on its target.

"Safety on this site, and for every man on this site is my job."

He paused and flicked the top page of his white Order Sheet quickly, without looking down on the form.

"The boy was drunk, like him under the influence of drugs. You never notice that?"

"The kid never drunk. Him just makes a simple mistake that other people here makes all the time, and you don't fire them all, do you?" Vandley contested.

Mr Davis was determined to show himself to be the boss of this site.

"Show me who else make that mistake what him just make? You see anybody else use a hammer when them suppose to use the puncher?"

He was not about to let the new comer challenge his authority.

"And you better off keeping you attention on your own job, man. The boy already walk off the site and the matter done so far as me is concerned. So everybody can go back to them work."

"All me a say is …"

The sentence was choked off prematurely by a further intervention by the foreman

"Is what? All you a say is what?" He completed the sentence started by Vandley.

The foreman continued, "If is your friend and it bother you fe see him go, then you can walk too, you know. Walk man. Follow him and walk to."

The foreman stood facing the two black workers standing nearest to Vandley.

"I have to make sure say this site safe. And if anybody drunk or drug up, them can't come here and work. You hear what I saying?"

"So you think say that because we is black people that we have to drug up and drunk?"

Vandley was also visibly angry at the accusation levelled in the direction of the three black workers standing near by.

"You a idiot, boss. Is where you come from?"

Vandley was left to defend the integrity of the group now standing around and showing their agreement by their body language if not by their words.

"You is a Jamaican as well and you want to treat black people like them is fool. You don't black too?"

Mr Davis didn't take kindly to being called an idiot, and he resented even more being accused of treating the black workers any more unfavourably than any other nationals. He didn't wait very long before making his gesture for Vandley to leave his site with some parting words.

"And if you or anybody else think say just because me is a black man too so you can take liberties, then you know where the road to the car park situated."

The show was now over and most of the workers on the building site must have eaves dropped on at least some part of the arguments. Vandley was on his way to the car park with his tools and overall. The hard hat was left on a small pile of hardened concrete for the foreman to collect. He was through with working for this and any other foremen who didn't treat black people with respect. After all, this was America and everybody was entitled to equal rights and justice under the constitution, even if they were Jamaican immigrants. The next two jobs also came and went quite quickly. He liked the driving job. Perhaps he could make his money as a courier driver. He would check out a few more contacts and see whether he could get into that line of work.

Chapter Eleven
Together Again

A brief return home to the island provided Vandley with a welcome break from the endless pressures of the Big Apple. Ron had married Lize on 27th August 1950. Following his retirement in 1987 from working at the Elkington Copper Refinery in Walsall they headed home to the island together for a final time. Ron had tarried almost thirty years in Britain with most of that time spent away from his wife and children. But they both loved their family and a way to reconciliation was found some eight years earlier. They survived the devastation of hurricane Gilbert a year after their return in 1988 when major areas of buildings and vegetation were swept away by the scale six storm. After calm had returned the family at home and abroad agreed to share the planning of the milestone Ruby Wedding Anniversary. This event would be a family celebration and the likes were never before seen in the district of Montpelier. The oldest children of Ken, Bibs, Earva and Vandley were the only ones born at the time of the marriage in 1950 and none was old enough to remember the occasion. There were no photos available to bear witness. All of the nine children and their grandchildren and a great grandchild would now be present as the vows were renewed. The full scale of the occasion would be planned in strict secrecy without the knowledge of the renewed bride and groom.

During the period of planning, a constant flow of teleconferencing took place between family members scattered between the island, Canada, the United States and England. All the trimmings and trappings of a family wedding were in place. There was an officiating minister, rings, bridal party, organist, confetti and Master of Ceremony for the reception. A Five-star hotel was booked for their one night honeymoon in the Bridal Suite. "You look nervous, Ron."

Denzil was just saying out loud what everyone else could see.

"Me no nervous, man. Me just can't wait till everything finish. Too much people is here."

"Don't worry about the people them, Ron. Everybody is here to see you and Lize tie the knot again."

Ron was often asked what he could remember of the original occasion.

"Boy, it was a long time ago now. That was in the 1950s and me mother and father never dead yet."

It was in Lize's home district of Cascade in Hanover, that they had got married.

"The church did full. Whole heap of people from Montpelier came over. Them boys who was already in Britain sent back money to me and them keep a big dance in the crossroad."

Ron didn't seem to recall much detail about how he was emotionally. He gave the impression over the years of being a man who was not afraid to show his emotions. The stag party was in full swing with a few crates of Red Stripe beer and Heineken being passed around to the guests invited mainly by Denzil.

"So you did cry, Ron?" Denzil's question was delivered with a broad grin and a hint of mischief. Ron had no intention to let the joke stick on him.

"You mad? What me fe cry for?"

Vandley joined in the ribbing.

"I bet you cry! I bet…"

Ron interrupted.

"No man, me never cry. Is only Lize one cry."

"And you never cry?" Denzil made a deliberate effort to emphasise the 'you' to Ron.

"No sir." Ron was determined to not lose this argument. He could at least be assured on the grounds that none of those present now was around back in 1950.

Lize had been persuaded to leave the comfort of her home by her daughters for the make do 'hen party'. The party of three merry sisters, nieces and family friends may have opened a bottle or two but they would have to get the tranquilliser out for anything more than a small drop of wine to pass Lize's lips. She was an avowed opponent of all things alcoholic but could just be swayed to make an exception on the day of her wedding. Ron on the other hand did not need any second invite at his stag night party on his veranda. When he finally agreed to retire to bed to rest before the break of the morning, eight or nine crates of beers and stouts had been emptied along with wines, brandy, white rum and the extra strong bootleg rum that locals gave the name 'John Crow Batty'. The roosters in the open yard had already begun to count down the hour in a simultaneous chorus of cock-o-doodle-do. When morning came, the skies were high and blue. It was shaping into a fine August day for a family wedding.

"Roland Norman Riggan, will you continue to take Sybil Eliza to be your lawfully wedded wife, to have and to hold, for richer or for poorer for as long as you both shall live?"

"Yes sir! I will."

"And do you Sybil Eliza, take thee, Roland Norman Riggan to be your lawfully wedded husband, to have and to hold, for richer or for poorer, for as long as you both shall live?"

"Yes, I will."

"Then with the powers vested in me, I now pronounce you man and wife, again."

The minister looked up from his open book. He peered over the rim of his dark metal-framed glasses. He anticipated the excitement from the open grins and smiles.

"Kiss the bride, Ron". Denzil led the chorus. Other people joined in.

"Go on, Ron, you may kiss your lovely bride."

The minister was only partly finished when Ron comically reached across to hold his wife and then laid an audible smacker on her lips. At that moment he could be forgiven for confirming to Denzil that this was also the way he had done it the first time around. He didn't look nervous and he was not crying. But they were both very happy in their special moment. They were legally married for forty-one years in fact. The road they had travelled since 27th August 1950 had at times been extremely rocky. They had been apart and also returned together. They could also add to the forty years of marriage another five years of courtship and starting a family together. The wedding pictures and video recordings captured the warmth and enduring love between them. The worse that life threw at them had been overcome and they could now stand in the company of their children, grandchildren, great grandchildren, family, friends and guests with pride and joy.

Barry was missing from the wedding and family reunion celebrations in Jamaica. He had returned to American from the island after a long stay of nearly twelve months while his application for US citizenship was being considered. He had expended much of his funds and he decided against returning to the island for the celebration. But perhaps if he had been presented with an opportunity to attend the wedding of Lize and Ron he might have turned down the offer. After all, it was not a secret within the family that of all her children, Lize had an especially fraught relationship with Barry.

Chapter Twelve

Deep South

The journey by Vandley to North Carolina was a welcome respite after the long drawn out accident insurance claim process. He took up the advice given by his sister. He collected a suitcase and boarded the bus heading south. The intermittent stops in the state capitals in New Jersey, Philadelphia, Baltimore, Washington and Virginia went by in the darkened blur of the night. When the bus took its stop at the bus station at down town Charlotte, Barry was waiting. It was the dawn of a new day and there was a new feeling of optimism for Vandley. He soon found another job in the building industry. After the accident he had made a personal pledge to give more of himself to God and after a few days of moving around with his younger brother he had noticed a sign giving direction to the Briar Creek Road Baptist Church. He was uncertain as to the exact location of the building but decided that he would give some attention to finding the right direction and maybe on Sunday morning, he would visit and see what it was like.

He reflected on the church he attended in the district of Montpelier during his youth. That seems a long time ago now and the island was far away. This was a different type of church.

The congregation was largely white with a loose sprinkling of brown or black people. But at least he thought the hymns were familiar enough, if song with less spirit and verve. And of course the Scriptures were just the same. He recognises the Psalm of David any day of the week and providing that it was being read in the English Language. The pace of the service was tranquil for his taste and he noted that in this church nobody smiles! But at least he had fulfilled his personal promise to venture into this American southern Baptist Church. He was a son of the Christian church but had drifted away from it on a tide of adult trial and pressures. He was a little surprised when the minister noticed him sitting at the very back near the exit door and walked over at some speed.

"Hi. And how are you today? You're visiting us?"

He didn't allow Vadley much time to provide him with any meaningful response.

"Yes. I'm a visitor."

"Well I'm sure you are," replied the minister.

"No. I mean I'm just a visitor."

"Oh yes. I've noticed. And you are welcome here. Everybody is welcome."

Vandley wasn't certain whether that required a further response. But he was glad to be made welcome, even in a round about way.

"We have a few black members here, already," the minister continued.

"Yes. That is very good, Reverend."

"And will you visit us again?"

"I will think about it, Reverend."

"Oh yes. And you can let us know if you would like to come back here to our little family church."

The minister's invite didn't quite feel wholehearted to Vandley. But it was a church. The nearest one to his house, and he did make that promise to himself that he would make the effort to start attending Sunday service. He felt warmer towards the church and to their style of worship after further visits over the next weeks and months. A few members were quite friendly and there were even a few additional black faces fitting into the mix of the congregation. They were now getting more use to his enthusiastic clapping of the hands and singing from the soul. He was no longer a total stranger amongst the members. But he noticed that there were some individuals there who preferred to not make eye contact nor share their Sunday greeting with him. He knew he would always be an outsider amongst them but he had long learnt that with God it mattered only that both the words of the mouth and the meditation of the heart needed to be acceptable to Him. He felt that his words were good and his soul was glad.

When Vandley headed south from New York to North Carolina in 1991 he hoped to make a new start to a life that had become punctuated by bad luck in love and business. But where as some of his failed enterprise may have been due to bad choice of business partners, he repeatedly failed to judge the true character of women. When he met Susan Eubanks, his first white partner, in Charlotte, North Carolina, there would be no need to wonder any further. This was quite easily a match made in heaven. But on earth, in the American South, there were a few human obstacles to overcome. When he had first met Susan, he felt slightly weary and hesitant about what people would say. He was conscious of himself as a black guy with a white partner. He was conscious that some areas in the traditional American Deep South had remained uncomfortable with mixed racial relationships. It took much effort before Susan convinced her family about the acceptability of the union.

He was more secured in the knowledge that his wife was a strong and resourceful woman. When they had first met at the Briar Creek Road Baptist Church in Charlotte, he was visiting the church and knew none of the members. Most were white Carolinians and Susan and her parents were longstanding members. He had always maintained a passion for worship and Christian fellowship. It was quite obvious to Vandley that some members of this congregation were not at all friendly and many seemed downright hostile to the presence of this stranger in their midst. He had already come face to face with racism and was not likely to give any credence to those around him who showed their hostility and ill will.

He had carried in his memory a previous occasion when living in Canada during the 1980s. It was in the middle of the harsh Canadian winter when he applied for and got a job with a lumber company. For five months in the winter, between November and March, he travelled to his place of work outdoors fully covered from head to toes. He spoke and interacted with work mates. Nobody ever bothered to ask whether he was black or white and everything went along swimmingly. When the fall arrived he didn't feel the need to wear all that warm clothing so the colour of his skin was revealed. Without warning, the foreman informed him that his services would no longer be needed. Naturally, he enquired as to why this was so because he could himself see the actual need for his continued service amongst the party. "These men don't want to work with blacks", said the foreman.

"But I have worked here with all of them for more than five months and never had any complaint", retorted Vandley.

"Well I'm sorry, Vandley, but I need all these good men, and if I keep you on, I will lose all of them."

That occasion was perhaps the first direct encounter that Vandley had with racism and bigotry. That same memory came back into his head as he sat at the back of the church in Charlotte. But amidst the hostile faces there was the gentle face of one young woman who he noticed. After several further visits to the church he begun to hold conversations with her and in time they became romantically involved. During the period of their courtship he was introduced to her parents and other family members. They were not as welcoming as Susan. He had often wondered whether their distaste was a consequence of their not knowing him or whether it was due to other reasons. As he got to know Susan better, he found her to be as brave and as bold as he had felt. The strength of her character was a very striking feature and it attracted him greatly. She was readily accepted and shown the unconditional love of his family. On the next occasion he visited the island he was more than eager to tell Lize and Ron and then his childhood friends about Susan.

"I always feel blessed, man. I really feel so." There was not hint of pretence in Vandley's demeanour or in his voice. He uttered the words because he believed every word. His boyhood friend Zeeke saw no reason for doubt. After all he had know Vandley since aged three or four.

"Well me think say you is right. I mean, when you did leave country and go to town you was just a little boy, then. And you did make it there, man. You really make it." Pausing to take another sip from his bottle of Red Stripe Beer, he continued, "Because you make it with the shop that you used to have." His eyes searched Vandley's face. "And is same way you go a Canada and you make it there too."

Dee filled the gap in Zeeke's words, " And the I never leave we out. True man. The I always come back ya. And the I bring things on here for I and I." The dread lock ruffled and was gently repositioned to the other side of Dee's head. "Is Jah bless the I. Selassie I know. A so it go."

"I have to feel blessed, man."

"Truly, dread. Is Jah love." Dee's voice sounded sincere, even if his eyes was starting to look red a bellow of smoke coming from his ganja spliff. The thin plaits of locks on his religiously uncombed hair was shaded by strips of grey.

"Boy, sometimes me used to think say some people just born with good luck. But is true Vandley, even if some of it was luck, you still make it. Yes man. You still make it."

When Zeeke paused again Vandley went quickly from the veranda to collect a further crate of beer from behind the neighbouring bedroom door. The company of boyhood friends had been chattering and drinking cold beer under an overhanging mango tree in the yard. Vandley was on a short holiday from North Carolina. He announced his recent wedding to his friends who still lived on the island. He would be leaving again in a few days, but while he was around his friends were always dropping by to spend some time over a bottle of Red Stripe.

"So how the wife stay Vandley? She nice?" Dee enquired.

"She very nice. She really gonna make me happy, man," Vandley replied.

Dee remembered some of the travails his friend had reported to him about New York. "Is Jah love, I, cause right now, I and I must know say the I find love. Yes I."

"My wife is really nice. And me have to love her right, and treat her right too."

"That is fe real, dread. The man must love the daughter right." After a further puff of grey smoke disappeared behind the dread locked hair, Dee returned to his subject.

"And the I must bring the daughter on yah so. So I and I can greet her, said way. Seen?"

Vandley was in agreement with his friend. "I'll bring her down here soon."

"The I must know say all a Miss Lize youths them is blessed, still. The whole a them. Jah know, rasta."

Zeeke was becoming unsteady on his feet from the white rum. He wanted to ask his friend about his plans for further children.

"So Vandley, you a go have more youths up a foreign?"

The company saw the funny side. Vandley obliged them with his answer.

"You have to wait and see guys. That is hard work you know brother." His broad smile was confirmation of his willingness to take up the challenge being clearly laid down by his old mates.

Chapter Thirteen

The Fruit of Reconciliation

Following their marriage, the fruit of their love was cemented by the birth of their only child, Angie. He was very pleased when the new baby was born. The quick scanning of the eyes over the child's narrow body had confirmed it was not his first son. She was beautiful. She was perfect. She was his daughter. Just for a brief moment his attention drifted away from Susan in the labour ward. This new baby will be the start of a new family that they will raise together. He knew that she was a first time mum but in his mind he had no doubt that she will be a fantastic mother. He already knew of her kindness and her love. Their new baby will receive a double portion of that love and kindness. He will never leave them alone. He would be there to share their lives always.

The rush of thoughts went through his head again and again. He thought about heading home to begin the assembling of the cot. He would call in at the local store for another pack of diapers. He wanted to do everything that he could to accommodate the new-born. Angie was given the name of her American grandmother. Vandley knew that the child would be accepted and loved by both her American grand parents.

The memories and experience of parenthood to his older children became vivid in his thoughts. He was there to support and protect them throughout their formative years until the relationship with their mother broke down. He had left the island for Canada during the mid-1980s and from where he continued to provide the children with financial support. It was during the time in Canada that he formed a new relationship and from this his fourth daughter Taataneisha was born. Her mother Hyacinth had other children before their daughter was born. The relationship did not become fully established but Vandley accepted his paternal relationship and provided his daughter with financial support.

The birth of Angie would provide a new opportunity for Vandley to share in the support and development of his child right from the start. He was very perceptive during the early years and formative stages. Between working hours he let his mind wonder freely about both his wife and child. He wondered whether he had performed the sterilising duties properly. The technical nuance of sterilising bottles was not the sort of thing that he was one hundred percent with. He was on much more certain ground with the heating of bottles to feed his daughter. On those occasions where Susan asked him for some help with burping and nappy change it made him feel useful and he looked forward to those practical things. He was a practical man. In his work he made practical use of his hands. He was looking forward to the moment when baby Angie begin to crawl around on the carpet and when he will be able to take her for a drive in the passenger seat of his truck.

The onset of spring was very welcome. He had already greased and checked over the lawn mower and soon the spurts of green shoots across the garden would be cut and raked away. Baby Angie was now just over a year old and was starting to find her feet, at least she did on the smooth of the carpet inside the house. Over the next four months to the end of the summer Vandley would attempt to spend as must time as possible in the company of his wife and daughter. As Susan joined him on the deck at the back of the house he looked closely at the face and hair of the child.

"Who do you think she looks like, Susan? I think she looks just like you. The same face and your smile too."

"Maybe a little bit, but I think she looks so much more like you, Vandley."

He continued to fix his gaze in the direction of the little girl.

"Come here, angel."

The broad smile exposed the white tooth and the slight gap in the centre of the upper row. His tanned skin was several shades darker than the lightly tanned hue of his daughter. Her hair was already dark and curly. It would soon be as long as that of her mother's. The brown eyes were deep with a tendency to wander involuntarily to either side as the head pivots sharply.

"I bet she will be very tall, Susan?"

"Do you think so Vandley, 'cause I'm not very tall; only five six. And you are only five nine or so." Susan surveyed the child further.

"She might be as tall as your mum though, or as your brothers."

"I think she will be a tall girl." Attending to his daughter with mock baby talk, "A bet you will. You will! Wont you? Wont you? You will 'cause daddy say you will!"

Whenever Vandley was at home with Angie and Susan, there was a surge of excitement. The child seemed to rush from one stage in her development to the next on a weekly basis. Before the start of winter several words were already clear. This encouraged him to introduce his daughter to some of the contents of his shopping bags. She was taught the history and the sweet taste of the ripened banana. There was a further lesson about the plantain.

"This is a plantain, Angie. It looks just like a banana, but it's different. And daddy will fry some for you and mummy." He made it his role to tell his daughter about all the lovely fruits on the island that he was familiar with as a young boy. His mind drifted back to some of his own memories of racing his friends to find the ripest mangoes. He was always amongst the winners in the search and find games they used to play. There weren't many tropical fruit trees in Charlotte or Raleigh. There was not the same freedom for a child to roam freely without the parents having to worry with fear of human predators. This was not the island and he was already aware that his daughter would need a strong will and determined character to overcome some of the potential challenges that will litter her path. When he was growing up, he was quite unawares of the hostilities he had experienced since he belatedly arrived in the States. He wondered whether a child might also be exposed to the same prejudices, even from familiar faces? But she won't have to worry because he would always be there to guide her path and offer her protection from all of that. Racial prejudice was nonsense. After all, he believed the word of his bible. All was created in the image of God. His spirit was not white or brown or black. He was a spirit of love and justice and peace. His daughter would not have to go through that nonsense. He would be there to see to it. He had been thinking of going back to the island during the next summer holiday. Angie would be out of elementary school and they could at last go to spend some time with grandparents Lize and Ron. Susan would take a break as well from her work that was now been done from home in order to be available to attend to Angie. He would also take the opportunity to talk to Lize and Ron about a couple of ideas he had been carrying around in his head. He had previously surveyed some of the grounds to the family home in Montpelier district with the intention of setting into motion the exploratory ideas for designing and eventually erecting a building for use as a commercial letting for holiday guests. It was an idea he had pondered over for at least a few years and the time was beginning to feel right for another look. If Lize were in agreement with the broad plan that he had sketched out then that would be a source of major reassurance. He was serious about the idea and he was of the intention to do something with it after he came back from speaking with his mother and father.

Chapter Fourteen

Disappearance in the Mist

The long and winding journey through the lives of Lize and Ron drew to its close on 31st July 1999 when a serious bout of illness led to her final departure from this life. Their life together had continued for more than fifty years through courtship and marriage. The number of Lize's days was seventy-six years. She had departed this world before any of her own children. When her oldest grand child, Melva, presented the eulogy of her grandmother's life it recognised the overwhelming contribution she had made as the backbone of the family they created together. She was fondly remembered as an enduring and steadfast matriarch who demonstrated the hands of fairness, a loving compassionate and generous heart. The full range and breadth of her life skills and abilities were recognised in tributes to her lasting memory, with Melva reminding the large final gathering thus,

> She was a constant source of encouragement to
> her family and to those who came into contact with
> her. She was a community person. Her passion
> to help others was well known. As a respected
> member of the community she was often called

upon to perform the duties of a banker, a lawyer, a councillor, an advisor, a teacher, a mother, a friend and a confidante. She would often write and read letters for members of the community who were unable to do so for themselves.

The loss of Lize to her family proved to be very difficult for Ron. Her days in the nest of the Riggan family were not without hard challenges but by her quite remarkable strength of character most of these were overcome in time. When tears were wiped from his eyes and the grave sealed, Ron withdrew to a state of deep personal reflection. He would remember his wife as the rock of his own life. He would give her the credit for rearing the family they had created together and wondered whether he given her as much love and support as he was able to give. Maybe, he thought, he didn't do right by her when he had first settled to a new life in England.

He recalled some episodes in his own life that he would have liked to erase completely from the annals of his memory. He recalled moments of her gravest anger and admits in his head and heart that he was wrong. He thought that maybe, if she had been married to someone else, who had a similar strength of will and personal determination she could have become a more fulfilled person. He clutched on to the many memories of their life apart and together as a new shower of tear soaked into his cheeks.

"Lize", his voice was just loud enough for himself to hear, "You gone left me, gal. Only me one left now. You left me by myself."

Ron looked around the bedroom he had shared with his wife. Her clothes were still present in the half-open wardrobe. He remembered her wearing the navy blue hat and white handbag to church. He fiddles uncomfortably with his fingers and hand, "What going to happen to me now?"

Ron did not regret the fact that the five years he planned to stay in Britain had multiplied six fold to thirty years. Having set off as a young family man in his early thirties, he was to return finally as a retired pensioner. Did he regret anything? Perhaps not knowing his children as they grew up on the island? He certainly felt the stirring of his conscience when he closed his tear filled eyes and recalled from memory the reaction of his wife to the affairs he had while they lived apart. He felt the need to whisper that he was sorry for hurting his wife. He had never stopped loving her. His life was completely intertwined with her memory and that was the most important thing for him. Now that she was gone, he found himself missing her even more than he could have expected.

"Me going to miss you, Lize. You know say you was the first and the last one for me. No one else for me but you." Ron responded to the good wishes he received from family and friends. The funeral was over now and he was determined to show everybody that he could continue his life after his wife.

In many respects the death of Lize was not a complete shock to the family. Members within the immediate family were already aware that for a period of five or six months she made several visits to the doctor with a long-standing complaint about breathing problems. She had complained of feeling a tightening of the chest following even brief strolls between the rooms in the house. It was accompanied by a permanent and deep-set cough that affected normal breathing. There was a feeling of breathlessness from even short walks. The doctor said the condition was at least in part due to her advanced years. The only clinical prescription was cough medicine and tablets for any breathing or physical discomfort. When the final hour came upon Lize she was comforted by her daughters on the island, Noreen and Bibs, with the minister of the local New Testament Church of God administering the final rites. She had lived a long and challenging life and was deserving of her rest.

Denzil was concerned about his brother Vandley. They had travelled down to the island from the United States. They were separated by two years and had grown up together.

"Vandley, you alright, man?" Denzil asked. He had noticed that his brother was especially distressed by the experience of losing his mother.

"Boy, I just can't believe she has gone from us, Denz."

"I know it is hard, man. It hard for all of us too, you know. But you know say the old lady would still like to see that we love her and we accept say she gone now."

"But it hard to accept Denz. Real hard."

Denzil was always close to his brother. They were separated by only two years in terms of age. Their own lives had been lived in close physical and personal proximity to each other.

"Vandley, Lize wouldn't want her death to leave you messed-up. She know say we a go miss her, man, but she know say we live close."

"We can't live so close without Lize, Denzil"

"But why not, man? Denzil repeated the question: "Why not?"

He could almost sense the presence of a deep despair overtaking his brother. He was drawn to him in a protective way. His right arm reached out and rested across his older brother's shoulder.

"Things will be alright, man. We will stick together. Things will be alright."

The family song played from a small recorder and a large huddle of bodies emerged together. Sounds on their voices drift into their cry and mourning. They accepted that the span of Lize's life was complete and they will return to their homes in various parts of the world with the collective memories of the mother and grandmother and aunt and friend who had now departed.

At age seventy-nine, Ron had entered a new millennium. He looked around the living room area of the house. A photo of he and Lize hung on the wall next to the television. She had never strayed far from his thoughts. He often sat in the long red leather upholstery chair on the veranda and just let his mind wonder back and forth on memories of his wife. He wondered whether his time would come soon. It was nice to hear talks about things that occurred during the course of the last century. In fact, he almost felt some entitlement to speak about many events to the children and young people who would visit him with parents and grand parents. His carefully timed interventions often followed a point of disputed fact relating to a well-known war or other event.

"Man, you hear them young ones talking 'bout new millennium, and them don't even know say if it wasn't for England, we wouldn't have no millennium?" The neighbour was averse to events of the Second World War. He continued to challenge of his younger challengers. "But is what you know 'bout history?" "You did know say is war have to fight to give we freedom to live right here so?"

He invited Ron to back up his facts. "You can tell them 'bout history Ron, 'cause you did live a England. Is no True, Ron?" The intervention was timely and Ron shared some of his own views about the world war. He was minded to tell his listeners about the role of Mr Churchill in England. They also had it from Ron that Adolph Hitler was a wicked German who had planned to kill all black people after he was finished killing Jews.

For a moment Ron didn't dwell on the memory of his wife. He could smile and share the wisdom of his years with a company of keen listeners. He knew that he would not be around too long into the new millennium but at the very least, he wanted to remind them that life was really short and the times would get even more dangerous for those still around after he was gone. It would be a further three years into the new millennium when it was time for him to say his final goodbye.

Ron had built up a huge memory bank with information about his family. He tried to recall the uncles and aunts by both his father Samuel and mother, Margaret. Memories of his parents' face were still held secured in the memory. He wondered just how old his father would be right now. He had died after Ron left for Britain in 1957. In his mind's eye he could see the old man, smoking on his beloved pipe. His physical statue was not more than five foot and one inch from sole to crown. Ron remember that even when Samuel had reached his own advanced years he was still quite active in moving about the yard and in attending to his animals. He was a man of jovial spirit. He lived as one with his five brothers and a similar number of sisters. The memory of his mother was still present and he recalled the round shaped face and blue patterned bandanna to partially cover the grey hair. He thought about the physical likeness between his mother and sister Lillian. When he came to England his sister Lillian was already there with her husband. His given name was James Ogilvie but he grew up with the nickname of 'Judge', due largely to a demeanour of seriousness and a stern manner devoid of any real humour. They had met during their late teens while working on the same commercial farm in the district of Cascade during the early 1940s. Judge and Lillian had never got children of their own and she made herself available to share in the care and upbringing of the children of her brothers and sisters. The family pet name of 'Mother' was eternally attached to her throughout her days.

Ron reflected on the brothers and sisters who had departed this earth ahead of himself. Already gone were Harold, Agnes, Thomas, Addy, and Gussy. They had remained on the island and never left with the rest who travelled to Britain. He would leave behind Nita, Dawz and Moodie. In England, he had lost Cyril, Joslyn and Lillian. He felt a tinge of regret that he had returned to the island and was unable to return to say his personal farewell. But at least, he thought, his brothers George, James, Elija and Lambert were all still alive in Britain.

Chapter Fifteen

Meet you in the Morning

The news of Ron's illness came to Vandley as quite a surprise. He was aware that his father had been feeling a little down in recent days and when he had telephoned to confirm his intention to visit, he had the sense that Ron was not at all enthused in the way of previous visits. There was some mention of having visited the doctor with Bibs or Noreen only recently. Maybe he was still feeling blue from being alone in the house so much of the time. But the doctor didn't say anything serious was wrong. He thought to give it a few more days and then telephone again and have another chat to Ron and see if anything had changed.

"Where are you Vandley? Its your sister Noreen from Jamaica on the phone." Susan placed the cordless phone on the dining room table. She was aware that he had gone to the phone and the sound of his voice trailed off as he quickened his steps and disappeared through a door into another room. He may have been gone for quite long. She wasn't sure. But she noticed the look of horror on his face from across the hallway. He was obviously upset.

"Vandley? What is wrong? Is something wrong? Is it Noreen?"

"Oh Ron died Susan. Just a little while ago. Noreen just rang me."

The confusion was still clearly printed on his face. The eyes were peeled back, open and then closed.

"I don't believe Ron he just died, Susan, and just like that?" The steps again hastened. He was quickly through the door and heading towards the truck. A turn of the ignition key and it was off the drive and heading down toward the bottom of the street. Susan had seen him upset by personal matters before and she would leave him alone for the time being. She knew he just needed a little time and space to begin to grieve the death of his father.

Two and a half years had passed when Ron had followed his wife into the sunset. The funeral service planned for Ron was put in motion very quickly. Noreen was the nearest in living around a third of mile away from Ron. She had been very saddened from losing her mother. Lize was a very good friend and confidant to her for as long as she was able to remember. As the child next to Barry she had always made the special effort to respond to Lize with respect and manners. Barry had proved a good foil for how not to behave with her mother throughout their formative years. It had pleased Lize that her youngest daughter never left the membership of the church. She was also pleased when Noreen took up a new post as aide to the local nurse immediately after leaving school. Noreen was too young to be held culpable for the breakdown in the plan to get all the children to Britain. The only significant disagreement they held as mother and daughter had stemmed back to her choice of a husband who was from Montpelier district. Lize held a view about just about every family in the district and she never reneged from the advice that it would be best to find partners whose family was from outside the district. By marrying anyone in the district she had forewarned that it would bring about the mixing of blood relatives and lead to strive between families with long standing grudges. She would not be overtly warm to William McNish but in time Lize came to accept that her daughter had married a good and descent man from the district. They were able to reconcile any differences in their contrasting opinion on the subject and shared many happy memories together as a family.

The relationship between Noreen and Ron was only begun when he retired to the island in September 1987. Her memory of him was stored from their previous meeting when he briefly returned to the island in 1968. She was still a schoolgirl at aged fifteen at the time. She remembered that he spoke with a soft voice and used words only sparingly. She had sent him many letters over the years while he was in England. Some of the things she had asked of him she received. He had sent some money to help with the cost of her wedding in 1972. She also remembered the new items of clothing he sent by parcel post on several occasion. The retirement years didn't get off to a good start either. They had returned less than three weeks when the shores of the island faced a severe battering from a tropical storm. Named Gilbert, the ferocity of the wind had decapitated the roof of the new house they had built in the district. She was their main source of contact and assistance in the midst of confusion and anger provoked by the storm and the response by the civil authorities. At the hour of his departure Noreen was at the ready to lead the planning and co-ordination of her father's funeral service until others alight and joined her. The wake singers celebrated in the style of traditional Caribbean rites and sentiments.

Suppose we don't Meet
Suppose we don't meet
Suppose we don't meet on the judgement day
Oh What a weeping, and mourning
Suppose we don't meet on the judgement day
(Traditional Jamaican Wake Song)

The memory of Lize was still fresh in Vandley's mind. During his most difficult times in Kingston and later in Canada and in the States, he had leaned heavily on the advice provided by his mother. The relationship with Ron was more a cordial friendship between two men who shared something of value. They both loved Lize. When Vandley had presented his mother with his self-styled plan to create a piece of history by planning the construction of a landmark guesthouse in the grounds owned by the family, he was discouraged by Lize, while Ron was quite prepared to listen to the idea. That plan never reached fruition in the end but Ron quite admired the sense of enterprise shown by his son. Vandley stood in the church during the funeral service to give a highly emotional address. He spoke in his usual rasping mixed American/Jamaican accent, 'Ron has gone. He wants you all to know that he loved you all very much.' He stopped to look up from the sheet of white paper held in his slightly nervous left hand before continuing, We don't know who is gonna' be the next one to follow Ron. That's why he ask me to tell you that you should start to live good with each other. Stop fighting with one another and be good neighbours.' He went into a rather personalised rendition of an old hymn:

I'll meet you in the Morning, Ron
By the bright riverside,
When all sorrows have drifted away:
Ron, I'll be standing at the portals,
When the gates open wide

At the close of life's long dreary day.

I'll meet you in the morning, Ron
With a 'how do you do'
And we'll sit down by the river
And with rapture "auld" acquaintance renew,
You'll know me in the morning, Ron
By the smile that I wear
When I meet you in the morning,
In the city build four squares.
I'll meet you in the morning, Ron
In the sweet by and by,
And exchange the old cross for a crown,
There will be no disappointments, Ron
And no one shall die,
In that land where the sun goeth down.

I'll meet you in the morning, Ron
At the end of the way,
On the streets of the city of gold,
Where we can all be together,
And be happy for aye,
While the years and the ages shall roll.
(Abridged from the Pentecostal Church Hymn: 'Ill
Meet You in the Morning)

In spite of the loss of Ron following on four years after Lize, the family did not feel cheated by their departure. Both had lived long lives by any measure and their mission in life was that of bringing up their children in a manner that reinforced a special trust and loving bond between family. They accomplished that mission and by reason of health and age the children accepted their time had come.

The family considered it fortunate that they could recall the premature loss of only one member. Floyd Kendrick Stewart was only twenty-three years old when he died in 1986. This came after many years of struggling to overcome a malfunction about the heart that was caused by an enlarged valve. It was a condition that had gone undetected for much of his childhood and youth on the island. As a baby Floyd and older sister Melva had returned from England in the care of Lize. Their mother, Bibs, remained in England with her husband before they returned to the central parish of Clarendon in 1970. After their grandmother left the island for England for the second time in 1979, both Floyd and then Melva also returned to join their grandmother. The heart condition was eventually discovered by the family General Practitioner but by then it was feared that it may have been too late to correct the problem. A prescribed course of special medication did not have any real effect and the family was deeply saddened by the premature loss of Floyd. The only other close relatives they had lost since that time had been for reason of age and failing health over a period of time. They could also be pleased that amongst their number, they had all outlived both parents.

Chapter Sixteen

Never be Lonely Again

"**C**ome over here, Angie, and say hello to your Aunt Noreen." The bright-eyed three-year-old responded to her father without hesitation.

"Hello, my name is Angie Riggan."

"Angie Riggan, you are a beautiful American girl, aren't you?" Noreen reached out to collect her niece from a standing position on the tiled veranda floor. This time Angie hesitated. She looked up towards her father. Vandley gestured his approval for her to go to Auntie Noreen.

"And what is that, auntie?"

"That is a humming bird. Have you ever seen a beautiful bird like that, Angie?"

The response was immediate. "Oh no, I've never seen any other bird like that one."

"Would you like to catch it?" Noreen took the hands of her niece.

"Oh yes! Help me catch it, Auntie Noreen."

Angie's legs were fully suspended in the arms of her Auntie Noreen while the fully lit brown eyes remained focused on the object of this adventure.

"Can I catch it now?"

The bird was already disturbed when a tentative reach of one arm was outstretched. A grab was not enough to trap the sharp reflexes of the island National Bird. The full expansion of the bird wings signalled its intention to move on to a safer feeding blossom.

When Vandley returned to his home in Charlotte with Susan and Angie he was still troubled by the loss of his father. It was a personal loss and the sense of void continued to linger in his thoughts for several days and weeks. Following the change over in the flight from Montego Bay to Miami, they took another flight to Douglas International Airport in Charlotte. He was tired but pleased to be home again. He had developed a deep cough. Tomorrow it would be Sunday and he intended to give church a miss just this once. Then it will be time to get back to work.

He thought the feeling of a severe Monday morning blues would soon go away. The temptation to make the phone call to the building site contractor was overwhelming. When the call was made he was told that the next job drywall wouldn't be ready for at least a couple of months. He had hoped that everything would return to normal in a few weeks. The trip back to the island for the funeral service of his dad was tiring physically and emotionally. Susan and Angie seemed to have settled down to their respective routines. Vandley continued to feel worse over the next week and made an appointment to see his doctor, who gave him medication for congestion. He continued to feel poorly. On Father's Day in America, Sunday, 15th June 2003, Vandley told his Pastor at Brier Creek Baptist Church that he wished to give a testimony. After the church announcements, Vandley went to the church podium and spoke to the congregation.

*"I don't know if you've ever been lonely before,
but I've had a rough week, a rough month and I
expect to have some further rough times ahead.
It has almost been four years since my mom
passed from my dad, and its like its broken
everybody's heart. Now my dad has followed her.
So, I know what it means to be lonely."*

Vandley cleared his throat and gave a rendition of one of his favourite songs.

> *Lonely days and lonely nights, filled with despair,*
> *Caused me to long for someone to care,*
> *Then I heard Christ say to me,*
> *"This promise I've made,*
> *Lo! I am with you now and forever, be not afraid".*

> *If you're longing for a friend, loving and true,*
> *Turn to the Saviour, he waits for you,*
> *He will do the same for you as he did for me,*
> *He'll never leave you, never forsake you,*
> *Trust him and see.*

> *Chorus*

> *I'll never be lonely again, never again,*
> *For I have opened my heart's door to Him;*
> *So I'll brush away the tears and forget my foolish fears,*
> *You'll never be lonely again, never again.*
> *You'll never be lonely again, never again,*
> *If you will open your heart's door to Him;*
> *So just brush away the tears and forget your foolish fears,*
> *You'll never be lonely again, never again.*

> *(Adopted: Author Unknown)*

The month of June had turned into July. Already the summer sun was giving off real heat and the fresh green grass surrounding the house had sprang to a good height. Vandley had set his armchair on the deck at the back of the house and the seat provided a source of physical comfort but did not stop the mental churning.

"How are you feeling, Vandley? Any better today?" Susan asked her husband.

"I don' know. I just feel tired. Its like I don't got no energy to get up."

"Would you like something to eat right now?"

"I'm not hungry, Sue. I just feel tired." Responded Vandley.

"Do you want me to make another appointment with the doctor, Vandley? You might have picked up a bad virus from the time we spent in Jamaica recently."

His eyes attended briefly to the look of concern on his wife's face. Perhaps he had picked up a virus on the island. He was conscious of the onset of a niggling cough that was causing some discomfort in the area of his body below the ribcage on the left side.

"Maybe I'll feel better in another few days. But if I don't start to feel good in my body, then I will go to see the doctor again."

The next visit to the doctor would follow when a further phone call to the building contractor became necessary. The doctor completed the routine check of heart and lung functions. The blood pressure test showed a normal reading. The pulse rate was steady but there were signs of some frustration in the breathing. It was too shallow. There will be a need for further tests and exploration. When the doctor communicated the delayed test result to Vandley in his office, they both felt an uneasy tension. The doctor had checked not once but twice to confirm the diagnosis of malignant cancer cells in the region of the left lung. There was a retention of fluid in the lung and this needed to be drained away. The nearest hospital was alerted to make available a room and the process to drain the fluid from the lung would begin.

Susan made a note of the telephone number in the hospital room before making telephone calls to her parents, Dr Bill and Angie Eubanks. She dialled the number of the building contractor and then turn to the long list of names on the page she had headed Vandley's family. The desperately sad news of Vandley's illness and diagnosis of stage four cancer of the lung was conveyed to the family by Susan. It was only a few weeks after the funeral of Ron back in Jamaica. Most family members receiving the news took it as an absolute shock. Susan fielded spontaneous questioning of the stage of the cancer. It was a heavy shock; unexpected and cruel. How could this be? The questions to Susan from different family members contacted were spontaneous.

" Is Vandley in much pain?"

She replied almost instantly, 'No, and he's resting much better now'.

"Are they sure about the diagnosis?"

"The doctors have been very thorough. They have checked and re-checked."

Susan was in a much better position than most to understand the process and reliability of the diagnosis. Her father was a medical doctor and she was employed in the field of radiology. She had no more reason to think that the doctors dealing with Vandley were not doing their very best. She was sharply aware that Ron had only been gone a few short weeks. She wondered how could such a threat hung over Vandley's life?

The diagnosis of Vandley's illness was especially difficult for the family because it came about the same time as Ron's youngest brother in England, Lambert, was fighting his own struggle against malignancy of the lung. The family held out in hope that Vandley would be able to do something that thousands across the world were failing to do each year. For one thing, they had all hoped that the malignancy could be held in check and that the medics would prevent further spreading and growth. But some of their optimism was also based on other reasons. Over the years the family had come to expect Vandley to perform incredible feats and escape acts. They held to the hope that he would dig deep into his physical reserves to somehow defeat this disease. And if all of these remedies failed they would all get down on bended knees to pray, day and night, and they would hold steadfast to the deep faith in the healing powers of God the Father.

Susan was hopeful that Vandley would get better and the encouragement offered by her father and friends at church added further reassurance. She knew the hospital very well. They were also her employers and doctors in the special unit had a good reputation for their clinical excellence. A full course of chemotherapy would be followed by radiology and in three to four months this problem should be overcome. It wouldn't be easy for any of them and during the course of the treatment he would need to be aided by a small canister of oxygen. The home environment was maintained in a state of cleanliness and comfort. Life would continue with church on a Sunday and work and school. They felt that there was really no reason to change anything within the home environment. It was important to reassure Angie that everything was really all right. Susan offered her comfort.

"Daddy is ill but he will soon be alright again, honey."

The family shared the most sincere hope that things could and would get better for Vandley. Ken held a conversation by phone with his brother. He may well have detected the anxiety in the voice and sought to reassure Ken of his determination to battle the cancer.

"I can't let this thing beat me, bro. The doctors said they could do something to stop it getting any worse. "

His optimism continued to show as he spoke.

" I still have things to do, big brother. I don't know how long it will take to beat it, but I will beat this thing."

This spirit of optimism served to galvanise the sense of hope that had still remained in all the family. Each day Vandley survived would inspire new optimism. When it finally dawned that there was not much that could be done a cloud of hopelessness set in. This condition quickly escalated beyond any medical control and when the end came the pain of sorrow was as a blunt instrument against the senses. Had Vandley needed a kidney, it would have been donated to him. If he needed bone marrow, this could be transferred to him. He could have had grafts of skin, litres of blood, any tissue or node. But cancer of the most aggressive kind cannot be thwarted, not even by the fire of prayer or the weight of love. When told by the doctors that they could do no more to prevent the growth and spread of the cancer, Vandley accepted that the end was nigh. He cried tears because he would be going away from the warmth and deep affection of his wife Susan. He knew he would not be around to protect and care for the youngest of his five children, Angie. He knew he was being taken away from the bosom of the family into which he was born and nurtured. He cried because others whom he knew loved and cared for him would be crying long after he had gone from their physical presence.

United in mourning, family members converged on North Carolina from their homes in Canada, the United States, England and the island among other destinations. The process of saying the final goodbye to Vandley was a difficult act. And as the sun set upon his life's journey the family had every reason to mourn in his memory. In tribute to the memory of Vandley they shared stories from his regrettably brief life. Juliene and her two older brothers, Chandale and Richie, were Barry's children, and they were close to their uncle. They had lived in an area of Charlotte near Vandley. The stories they shared seemed to capture the enduring love and kindness.

" When we were leaving Jamaica for the States, Uncle Vandley was there to help us to get ready. It felt like it was only yesterday", continued Juliene.

"He was wearing a white shirt with black stripes; white pants and some white shoes. He was laughing and acting crazy as usual."

Juliene's oldest brother Chandale could also recall from memory.

"When we got to New York that first time, he came over to the house where we lived. He always came over to the house to see how we were doing."

The brothers and sister shared a smile in genuine love for their uncle and continued, "He was again telling us jokes and playing games with us. He would make us laugh so hard, sometimes tears would just roll from our eyes."

Barry also shared memories of time enjoyed with his older brother.

"I always saw Vandley as my family hero. He was the only one in the family with practical skills. The man could build you a house if you could supply the material"!   Barry recalled an occasion when he was about to throw out his son Richie from his house. Before taking his drastic action, Barry went to seek the opinion of his older brother. The response was not quite what was expected.

"I used to go to work early mornings and finish the day at eight or nine o'clock. Vandley worked in Charlotte and would come to my house even when I was out", he recalled. For about a week I never went around to the back of my house. But after I had my chat with Vandley, I was home one day and heard a hammering sound. I couldn't believe it when I went around there!"

Vandley was present round the back of the house, and had converted the outhouse into a makeshift extended bedroom for his son. Barry was then advised to throw Richie out, but not onto the street but into the outhouse instead. With that practical intervention came a personal pledge by Vandley, that he would keep an eye on Richie.

Wakes and funeral services in the Caribbean are very emotive and expressive affairs. Traditional folk songs will come tumbling out with renowned wake singers holding centre stage. Drum beat and make shift musical instruments are guaranteed to enchant and entertain up to the eve of a family funeral. These affairs are quite special on Caribbean islands such as Jamaica. It was not a tradition that had made any impact in the leafy suburbs of Charlotte in the American South. In mourning, the family continued to express their love for Vandley through rendition of songs during the service of thanksgiving at the local Baptist church at which he was an active member. They shared in the reading of scriptures, tributes, eulogies and prayer.

They were reminded throughout the funeral service of the positive impact made by Vandley during the time living in Charlotte. Friends and strangers eulogised about the kindness and assistance offered to them by Vandley. Their moving tributes captured the genuine spirit with which he had approached life.

"In a world where many people pretend and wear masks, his openness and honesty was a rare treat", said a member of the local church.

Another told the congregation, "If I could have taken the cancer away from him, I would have done that for him".

In singing tribute, we were reminded that God's Peace would be with Vandley until we would all meet again in a Heaven, without disease, pain or death. The minister leading the service encouraged the family to 'tell the story of Vandley's life to his children, so that they would know what a good man their father was'. Vandley had already done his own crying. He was gone but would never be forgotten.

Chapter Seventeen

Gone but not Forgotten

The skies above Charlotte in North Carolina were clear. The two furniture removal trucks parked in the drive carried the neatly hand painted words: *Riggan Delivery Service*. Barry always waited until the quiet of a Sunday morning before he clear the vehicles and prepare for any work on the order books for the following week. He had been in this business for many years since taking a job as delivery van driver for a Korean family in Brooklyn, New York. They had been in the green grocers trade in the city over two generations. Barry was one of the two van drivers they had employed in addition to their youngest son. They liked his honesty and they could rely upon him to be available at anytime for the delivery of orders to clients and the pick up of new stocks.

The family had settled in Charlotte, North Carolina when they first landed in the United States as refugee from the Korean War with America in the early 1970s. The husband had recently died and his widow decided to return closer to the remainder of her family in Charlotte. She had told Barry of her decision and gave him the assurance that if he was minded to make the move south, them his job would be guaranteed. After thinking about the proposition, Barry agreed to the offer and he also relocated to the area. It was through that line of work and contacts that he graduated to establish a delivery business of his own in the furniture removal trade.

There was another quiet thought of Vandley in his head. It was usually at this time in the morning before church that he would put in an appearance at Barry's house. He called around to see how they were all doing. When there was any special event on at the church Vandley would invite the entire household to come along to the service with him. Chandale and Juliene were more likely to oblige their uncle and put in an appearance if only occasionally. Barry and Richie had never taken up the invitation. There was a tangible void in their lives. Barry thought of his brother as a kind and helpful man. He had been present to provide him with support when they lived in New York. Barry recalled that Vandley had provided his children with clothes when they first arrived from the island. He remembered his brother coming to the house with large bags of grocery to supplement and replenish their decreasing stock. There were the occasions when he had arrived in the cab to take the children to school on a Monday morning. There were the times when he collected them and waited on them. Barry walked to the shed at the back of the house. The extension build by Vandley had saved his son Richie from sleeping on the streets of Charlotte. There were just too many memories for him to hold onto.

"Up to now I still find it hard to believe that me brother gone from us. The man was not even old. Just about reach fifty. But fifty is not anything now a days? Ron did live until him was eighty odd. And them said we grandfather Samuel lived until him was around seventy."

There was a pause in his thought as he collected his brush and buckets from the shed. "So the man should a live for at least another twenty five years."

That thought was caught up in the moment as Barry dwelled on the unspent years. The years were not fulfilled and so in his mind, they were lost to his brother.

The flow of the water into the bucket from the kitchen sink was slow enough to leave the mind still wondering about his brother. He now had in his thought an image of his niece Angie. Her innocent smile. The sharp gaze from the light brown eyes.

"But how Susan and Angie going to cope now without Vandley? Is him who was them provider and them protector. Him was the heart of them family. How them a go cope now him gone?" A slow nod of the head in answer to the questions flickering around inside his head was the answer.

"Angie is only a baby. She was only four years old. She can't yet know about her father. How she a go remember him properly?"

The repetitive pushing and pulling motion of the brush was followed closely as his thoughts of the brother he loved the most scurry around in his head. The waste collected in the vehicle from the previous day's collection and delivery orders was the usual compilation of dried leaves from the shoe and strips of paint and polish. Parts of the plastic bags and brown paper bags that were usually shed from the packaging and parcels delivered alongside the heavy furniture of tables and chairs, fridge, cookers and sofa beds. In his mind he hoped that he would continue to be available for Susan and Angie. They are Vandley's family. They are his family. They would always be a part of the Riggan family.

The Children and Grandchildren of Ron and Lize Riggan

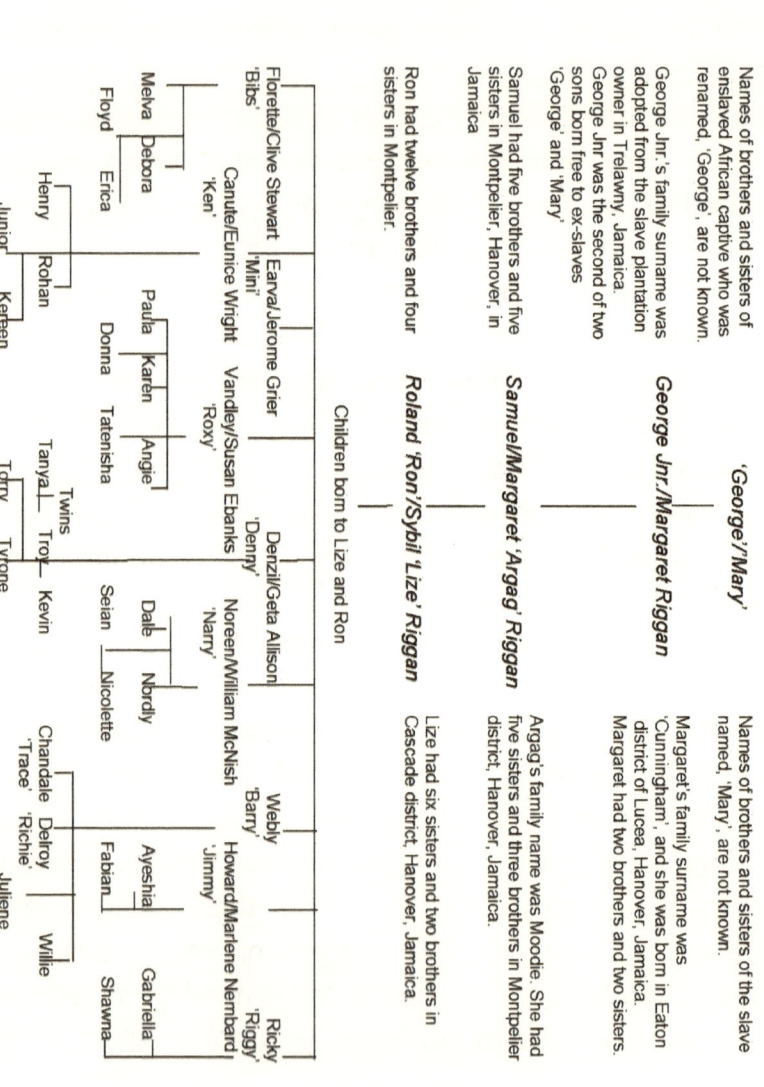

Names of brothers and sisters of enslaved African captive who was renamed, 'George', are not known.

Names of brothers and sisters of the slave named, 'Mary', are not known.

'George'/'Mary'

George Jnr.'s family surname was adopted from the slave plantation owner in Trelawny, Jamaica. George Jnr was the second of two sons born free to ex-slaves 'George' and 'Mary'.

George Jnr./Margaret Riggan

Margaret's family surname was 'Cunningham', and she was born in Eaton district of Lucea, Hanover, Jamaica. Margaret had two brothers and two sisters.

Samuel had five brothers and five sisters in Montpelier, Hanover, in Jamaica.

Samuel/Margaret 'Argag' Riggan

Argag's family name was Moodie. She had five sisters and three brothers in Montpelier district, Hanover, Jamaica.

Ron had twelve brothers and four sisters in Montpelier.

Roland 'Ron'/Sybil 'Lize' Riggan

Lize had six sisters and two brothers in Cascade district, Hanover, Jamaica.

Children born to Lize and Ron

Florette/Clive Stewart 'Bibs'
Melva
Floyd
Debora
Erica
Henry
Rohan
Junior
Kereen

Earval/Jerome Grier 'Mini'

Canute/Eunice Wright 'Ken'
Paula
Karen
Angie
Donna
Tatenisha

Vandley/Susan Ebanks 'Roxy'
Twins
Tanya
Troy
Kevin
Tony
Tyrone

Denzil/Geta Allison 'Denny'

Noreen/William McNish 'Narry'
Dale
Nordly
Seian
Nicolette

Webly 'Barry'

Howard/Marlene Nembard 'Jimmy'
Ayeshia
Fabian
Gabriella
Shawna

Ricky 'Riggy'

Chandale 'Trace'
Delroy 'Richie'
Juliene
Willie

132

Some Common Jamaican Words

Jamaican Words	Loose Standard English Translation
Coulda	Could have
Cum Ya	Come here
Dutty	Dirty
Fam-bly	Family
Gal	Girl
Go'wa	Go away
I and I	Myself
Jah	God
John Crow	Crow
'Memba	Remember
Mi	Me
Mim	Mum
Moggotty Bush	Moggotty Estate
Mom-pelier	Montpelier
Me naa look nobody	I am not looking for anybody
No sah	No sir
Nuff	Many
Oonu	All of you
Oofa	Whose
Pickney	Child

Jamaican Words	Loose Standard English Translation
Stove	Cooker
Tek'way	Take Away
Tryall Bush	Tryall Estate
Tun Off	Turn off
You fe go	You should go

About the Author

Born into a migrant Jamaican family, R. George Riggon started out on a personal quest to trace the historical movement and roots of his own family in searches that involved the use of historical records of births, deaths and marriages in Africa, Jamaica, USA, Canada and Britain. A desire to explore and share the rich source of historical information on African and Caribbean family genealogy between as many people as possible was the main motivation behind these works.

The author was raised and educated in England. He attended the University of Central England in Birmingham and Warwick University where he obtained a first degree in Sociology and a Masters in Race and Ethnic Studies respectively. Postgraduate training in research and management forms the basis of his professional work in public and community service sectors.

His two books: 'Living As a Riggan' and 'The Love of a Father, A Mother and A Son' celebrates the importance of family as an essential source of support and inspiration for present and future generations. Their publication also coincided with the bicentennial year since slave trading between the continent of Africa and the European controlled colonies of the Caribbean was ended in 1807.